Coping with Cancer

Coping with Cancer

Avery D. Weisman, M.D.

Professor of Psychiatry
Massachusetts General Hospital
Harvard Medical School

Principal Investigator, Project Omega
Department of Psychiatry
Massachusetts General Hospital

McGraw-Hill Book Company

New York   St. Louis   San Francisco   Auckland   Bogotá   Düsseldorf
Johannesburg   London   Madrid   Mexico   Montreal   New Delhi
Panama   Paris   São Paulo   Singapore   Sydney   Tokyo   Toronto

NOTICE

Medicine is an ever-changing science. As new research and clinical experience broaden our knowledge, changes in treatment and drug therapy are required. The editors and the publisher of this work have made every effort to ensure that the drug dosage schedules herein are accurate and in accord with the standards accepted at the time of publication. Readers are advised, however, to check the product information sheet included in the package of each drug they plan to administer to be certain that changes have not been made in the recommended dose or in the contraindications for administration. This recommendation is of particular importance in regard to new or infrequently used drugs.

Library of Congress Cataloging in Publication Data

Weisman, Avery D
     Coping with cancer.

     Includes bibliographical references and index.
     1.   Cancer—Psychological aspects.   2.   Cancer—
Social aspects.   3.   Adjustment (Psychology)
I.   Title.   [DNLM: 1.   Neoplasms—Psychology.
QZ200.3 W428c]
RC262.W44   616.9′94′0019   78-14906
ISBN 0-07-069009-X

COPING WITH CANCER

1 2 3 4 5 6 7 8 9 0   DODO   7 8 3 2 1 0 9

This book was set in Times Roman by The Total Book (ECU/BTI).
The editor was Orville W. Haberman, Jr.; the cover was designed by John Hite; the production supervisor was Jeanne Selzam.
R. R. Donnelley & Sons Company was printer and binder.

Those who are born too soon do not know
the glories of the future, but are spared
agonies yet unknown

Contents

Foreword

In the twentieth century cancer has assumed new dimensions as a human experience. The shift in life expectancy from 47 years at the turn of the century to 71 years in 1971 has been accompanied by an increase in sheer numbers of people with malignant disorders. Over the same span of years cancer has also shifted from being more than simply a dreaded human problem. It has become a target for the application of science and technology to its eradication.

For a variety of reasons changes in the new century have made it possible for more people to have cancer and to live with cancer for longer periods of time. Concurrently these social and technological changes have contributed to an objectification and depersonalization of provider-patient relationships as large complex systems evolved for the delivery of patient care services. Increasingly, coping with cancer has become a medicosocial as well as a personal process with the human concerns of people with cancer easily becoming secondary to the goals of scientific research and oncologic therapy.

This book is a timely reminder that science does not have to exist apart from humanistic values and concerns. Avery Weisman is one of those rare human beings whose writing conveys a dual commitment to the importance of scientifically grounded knowledge about cancer and the need for interpersonal transactions that respect the integrity and worth of the person. The concepts developed here are a thoughtful amalgamation of the results of his work as a behavioral scientist and his thoughts about intervention undoubtedly influenced by his contacts with cancer patients as a practicing psychiatrist.

The book is organized around a central theme that coping with cancer is simultaneously an intrapersonal and interpersonal process ongoing in nature and altered by changes in the person and the situation. In a series of ten chapters Weisman describes the nature of coping as it has been observed in cancer patients and relates these findings to some principles for action aimed toward helping people to achieve completeness in their lives. He examines in some detail the relationship of coping to hope and denial, the types of strategies that comprise the coping process, and some ways of predicting which individuals are likely candidates for high emotional distress and ineffective coping.

Applying the concept of staging to psychosocial responses and adaptations, he proposes an approach for evaluating morale in relation to the clinicoanatomical stage of the cancer and recommends some "best times" for initiating action on behalf of the person. He discusses the influence of provider-patient communication patterns on a patient's sense of trust and confidence in others and proposes some specific ways by which other people can assist a person with cancer to achieve an appropriate death. His chapter on countercoping as an approach toward effective intervention with cancer patients offers valuable insights into the difficult nature of being truly a helping person.

Anyone concerned with the complexities of living and dying with cancer should find this book an important reference. For practitioners in oncology the value is threefold. It contains a wealth of information about human behaviors in response to living with and around cancer. It provides a useful set of guidelines for recognizing the special vulnerabilities of people with far advanced disorders. It provides direction for taking action that promotes and supports positive coping behaviors in response to a highly stressful situation.

Jeanne Quint Benoliel, R.N., D.N.Sc.
School of Nursing
Department of Community Health Care Systems
University of Washington, Seattle

Preface

Some day, current theories and practices in tumor therapy will seem as obsolete as the remedies in a textbook of 100 years ago. Quaint and sincere as those outmoded concepts now seem, it is wise to remember that they guided generations of physicians who treated afflicted patients. Both doctors and patients managed as best they could. We are no different. After all, 100 years is scarcely a moment as time is measured. We recall that anesthesia was still novel; histological diagnosis of cancer was almost an innovation; radiation, chemotherapy, and most diagnostic measures common today were unimaginable.

Physicians and nurses of a century ago were probably no more or less humane and dedicated than our contemporaries. While improved technologies and specializations tend to compartmentalize medicine, technical triumphs do not mean ethical bankruptcy, nor does compassion flower only in the soil of ignorance. There are always shortcomings, and none of us is a stranger to failure. Consequently, it is not unreasonable to expect that, in years to come, comprehensive care of cancer patients will improve along with better methods of diagnosis and treatment.

Too often today, "comprehensive care" is limited to multimodal attacks upon the tumor itself. The patient is almost a bystander in the struggle to control this insidious collection of diseases known as "cancer." Too often also, even very advanced treatment is routinized by complicated protocols, or simply carried out according to institutional preference. Special rehabilitative programs regarding psychosocial needs and problems are secondary, receiving at the most a friendly gesture or kind comment, but scarcely a clasp of collaboration.

I do not advocate a subspecialty of psychosocial oncology. But cancer patients do have special coping problems that are shared with no other group, and therefore merit careful, systematic investigation and, sometimes, intervention. At the present, however, there are few clear pathways through these thickets of social and emotional complications. Nurses, social workers, physiotherapists, and other specialists who work assiduously day by day with patients and families are often acutely aware of these issues. Busy as they are, some physicians also recognize that after somatic treatments have ended, coping with cancer has scarcely begun.

In this age of medical spectaculars, it is only natural to admire the accomplishments of physicists, engineers, computer scientists, cellular biologists and so forth. Scientific research is in the forefront of progress. But let us not minimize clinicians and investigators who deal with individual patients, their problems, and families. From ancient times, man's fate has been the measure of all things, even of stars in the heavens. While mankind may not always have benefited, medicine has tended to follow the values esteemed by society at large. We are no different today in what we do and hold valuable. Like true scientists, we seek to measure just about everything possible, but many of the things that endow life with quality and competence elude computerization. We are, therefore, obliged to work with both measurements and with meanings that cannot be enumerated. We continue to look for principles to guide what we do. Otherwise, medicine is simply an exercise in empiricism and tradition.

Many social ills impoverish contemporary life. There is no greater aspiration for medicine than to help improve the life we have and want to hang onto. But simply to extend survival with one technological device after another would be empty and futile, unless we also heed human problems and learn how to cope with them. Cancer is a human problem. Psychosocial studies in cancer are but a sign of this vision.

Cancer is always newsworthy. From public health warnings about carcinogens to cell studies, tumor enzymes, and disease prototypes, the public and profession are bombarded by the roar of the "fight against cancer." Local skirmishes are reported, suggesting that total victory is imminent. Bulletins are issued, as if from a battlefront, quoting experts, like generals, saying, "Give us the funds and public support, and we shall not fail."

Public education and private attitudes about cancer are often at two poles, neither of which serves the cancer patient very well. At one extreme, emphasis is put on early diagnosis and prompt treatment. This viewpoint can hardly be disputed, except that early detection is not always possible, nor does it mean catching cancer at an early stage. Moreover, early diagnosis and prompt treatment are not a promise of absolute cure. Nevertheless, some patients are lulled into premature security, as if cancer treatment were quick and easy. The other extreme, however, is more pernicious and demoralizing. It perpetuates a tragic and absurd canard that cancer is the deadliest of diseases, and that its diagnosis is tantamount to a death sentence.

Meanwhile, the quiet search for better understanding seldom makes headlines. Psychosocial studies never draw much attention, even if the need for continued care of cancer patients is profound. Nevertheless, the human side of cancer is not irrelevant. Nurses, social workers, pastoral counselors, a few psychologists, a rare psychiatrist, and a scattering of physicians carry on the tradition so eloquently exemplified by Sir William Osler and Dr. Roswell Park.

For the cancer patient and family, there is nothing of greater magnitude besides cure itself, than how to cope best with problems, to understand aberrant behavior, to tolerate besetting distress through weeks, months, and even years. Indeed, uncertainty itself is a coping problem.

Until now, we have had to rely on the good will and improvisations of professionals who, understandably enough, lack coherent appreciation of the principles underlying the coping process. Extrapolations of professional expertise into the psychosocial domain have not provided adequate guidelines or directives, but at present, enough information has accumulated through research and application to justify a more systematic approach to problems of coping with cancer. These problems are quite different from studies of how cells become cancerous. However, I emphasize that while information is certainly better than conjectures and speculations based on a few cases, today's guidelines, like medical practice of 100 years ago, may be tomorrow's misconceptions.

Experience, of course, is the name we give to our mistakes. There can be no reliable information without an appropriate corresponding conceptual structure. Theories and hypotheses come together and provide a basis and an impetus for further research and rational care. Suppositions help no one. What are required are data gathered from many cancer patients with different types of cancer at various stages over an extended period. It is, fortunately, no longer justifiable to cover ignorance with generalities, even those sanctioned by tradition.

There is certainly no lack of literature about the biology of cancer. In the past two decades, an enormous literature of thanatology has also accumulated, much of which deals with cancer deaths—as if no one died of anything else. Psychosocial research in cancer has suffered from limitations in study groups and of working methods. Yet, understandably, patients and families want clarity, direction, and precision in coping with cancer and its vicissitudes. Admittedly, there are probably also just as many families, patients, and physicians who feel that psychosocial interventions are wholly superfluous or irrelevant.

Until cure is certain, coping with cancer remains a critical problem. *The diagnosis of cancer is not the same as being a cancer patient.* This distinction is often overlooked, because the plight of being a cancer patient is rarely investigated in depth. While we can, legitimately, wonder how deep is depth, for the individual patient statistics and histology are remote and academic. For that individual, there is only one consideration: "What about me?" A fraction of 1 percent still refers to people.

In a sense, having cancer is being had by cancer. Few know how firm that grip can be. "Something must be done about it" is a demand for better coping. The "best" patients believe at the outset: "I must cope with it, with whatever help is available."

What is a cancer patient? If one attends tumor conferences and witnesses the entrances and exits of silent patients, sitting or lying in various positions better to expose themselves for cursory observation, it is all too evident that the patient *is* the cancer, and very little more. Nevertheless, a cancer patient is a person who was generally well before being afflicted with a dreaded diagnosis, regardless of symptoms. The diagnosis also reorients a patient, creating a special relationship with a physician, a cadre of doctors, or an institution. From a physician's viewpoint, a good patient is someone with a curable illness, who cooperates fully, responds promptly, makes few demands, and recovers with minimal residues and maximal appreciation. But what of the chronically ill or incapacitated cancer patient who responds only up to a point? What of cancer patients who may not recover at all? Does this not also impose a special burden on professionals? Leaving aside the unconscionable physician who abandons patients, the most skilled and dedicated doctor may find himself committed to treatments which are, by definition, less and less effective or promising. Doubt and uncertainty befog the doctor-patient relationship.

The medical plight of cancer is not, therefore, confined to the patient. Coping with cancer and its ramifications is an ever-present necessity, from diagnosis on for everyone. Contrary to public and somewhat professional assumptions, most cancer patients do manage to cope very well. But others do not cope well, and become vulnerable to a variety of problems.

This book is the result of systematic inquiry into how cancer patients cope or fail to cope with issues related to their illnesses. These are, of course, psychosocial issues which emerge from the medical plight. I intend this book to be a more discursive, yet organized, companion volume to more technical research reports, published over many years. These articles have dealt with various aspects of liaison psychiatry, thanatology, and, more recently, the plight of newly diagnosed cancer patients. That there is a difference in how cancer patients cope is axiomatic, because, sick or well, people think, feel, and behave in somewhat unique ways, depending on what happens to them and how they dealt with earlier problems. Nevertheless, coherent observations can be made, and from these, principles derived.

Mere inquiry is not enough. Patients and families want practical and immediate help with psychosocial problems, even if such help is initially spurned. Only by studying how people cope from the onset, however, can we understand later complications. This truth emerged clearly from our earlier studies of the preterminal and terminal phases of life.

Psychosocial cancerology is barely in its infancy. I must use this term, instead of the more formal "oncology," to include the patient, and not merely the study of tumors. In some respects, we already have more knowledge than is generally used. In other ways, we do more than we fully understand or are able to formulate clearly. Cancer patients make it very apparent that continuing care involves much more than physical rehabilitation, prostheses, job counseling, friendly support, home nursing, or hospices.

Progress in medicine generally can be traced to two principal sources, other than through the day-by-day work of enterprising investigators and practitioners. One source comes from better understanding of the rationale behind what professionals are already doing empirically. This means that useful concepts and productive theories are distilled from the crude extract of daily prescriptions. A second source has often been the work of an informed, inquisitive outsider. His very distance provides for a perspective not available to those who are wholly immersed in a field and imbued with traditional viewpoints.

Just as the day of the solo practitioner is rapidly ending, no one does research in absolute solitude, without the help of devoted associates. Psychosocial medicine, in particular, is multidisciplinary in concept and in practice. Therefore, I cannot convey sufficient indebtedness to the people with whom I have worked closely during past years, especially those engaged in Project Omega. Our mutual goal has been not only to understand the latter stages of life, but to formulate principles of coping and vulnerability that pertain to the *completeness* of life. To me, completeness is what is signified by *Omega*.

J. William Worden, Ph.D., has been coinvestigator and research director of Project Omega from its inception. He has vigorously insisted on separating facts from myths, and on not being lured by speculations without substantiating evidence. Dorothy Wingquist, M.S.W., and Catherine Sampson, M.S.W., along with Jane Calhoun, M.S.W., during an earlier phase of our study, have been the first line of contact, as well as the agents of continuing alliance with patients and families. They carried the enormous burden of gathering data and comforting patients who were, in some instances, followed for months and years. Mrs. Joan Griffin has made all our projects run smoothly at every point, helping to compile information as well as assisting with this and other manuscripts.

The work on which this book is based has been supported by the National Cancer Institute, Division of Cancer Control and Rehabilitation (CA-14104). Thomas P. Hackett, M.D., Chief of Psychiatry at the Massachusetts General Hospital, has never faltered in his friendship, encouragement, and suggestions.

It is no small matter for the cancer staff of a large teaching hospital, busy with its own work, to allow us to interview, assess, and follow cancer patients under their care. Ordinarily, few of these patients would have been referred to psychiatrists, social workers, or psychologists. Because our aim has been to sample consecutive patients who first arrive at the hospital with a primary diagnosis of cancer, confidence in the principal investigator, accrued over many years of affiliation, has sometimes outweighed belief in the relevance of psychosocial procedures. I am profoundly grateful, but I also know that many physicians privately acknowledge that tumor treatment without heeding the host is unacceptable practice. I am deeply aware that each of us tries, in his or her special way, to uphold standards of excellence that this hospital has exemplified for generations.

Avery D. Weisman

Coping with Cancer

Chapter 1

Hoping Is Coping

The dark truth shadowing the fullness of a good life is that hazards surround us at all times. None of us is exempt. Among these daily dangers is the possibility of a chronic or incurable illness, of which cancer seems to be the prototype.

The main business of hospitals is diagnosis and treatment of disease. For many patients, however, illness is but a slight inconvenience. They recover rapidly, and go on about living with scarcely an interruption. For others, especially cancer patients, diagnosis is only the beginning. This does not, of course, mean that the diagnosis of cancer is an automatic death sentence, as so many unjustifiably fear. Rather, it is testimony to the perseverance and courage of cancer patients who must cope with a disease in which treatment is often prolonged and very uncertain.

Cancer is not just another chronic disease. It evokes many of the deepest fears of mankind. Despite assiduous, skillful, and intelligent treatment, it can spread throughout the body. It can also spread into social and emotional domains, drastically disrupting families and challenging the very values that make life worth living.

1

IS COPING POSSIBLE?

A surprisingly large number of cancer patients seem to cope very well with illness, treatment, secondary problems, and even with uncertainty itself. Our frail bodies, always poised precariously between disaster and disease, have a strong sense of survival that helps us accommodate to the unexpected. It is, at times, even somewhat miraculous to observe how well patients withstand the plight of cancer, while preserving a hopeful spirit. Their example is the theme of this book: how cancer patients at various stages of illness manage to cope and sometimes fail to cope with psychosocial and physical adversities.

I do not propose to write a how-to book that requires nothing of the reader and offers panaceas in return. On the other hand, I have found no adequate, comprehensive guide for coping with cancer that is based on substantial psychosocial research and clinical studies stretching over time. Patients, families, physicians, social workers, nurses, and other professionals are aware of the many dimensions of cancer. But most books about the very personal side of being a cancer patient are just that, and it is therefore difficult to generalize about specific situations. Some survivors who have lost a spouse, parent, or child, spurred by their own need to cope, have written memoirs of touching eloquence.[1,2,3] A few cancer patients also offer their own experiences as a guide.[4]

I believe that the scope of psychosocial distress is far greater than ordinarily realized. Patients who are happily regarded as "well-adjusted" have subclinical problems and emotional distress that persist long after the cancer has come under control. Nevertheless, many physicians minimize this aspect of cancer care. Their attitude, however, is somewhat paradoxical. On the one hand, psychosocial investigation is thought to be too speculative to be scientific. On the other hand, structured assessments and systematic evaluation of coping are deplored as being too detached to be practical and to help those in need.

While this book is but an elementary prologue to psychosocial cancerology, I offer a combination of the practical and the investigative. Thus, it may be useful to patients as well as professionals, in that I have sought general principles that might be applied to specific situations. I am deliberately not engaging in polemics about the causation of cancer, but rather make a disciplined effort to clarify the kinds of problems that cancer patients deal with, and how they do it.

Good will, compassion, common sense, tact, and honesty are precious ingredients of medical care that are always in short supply. But none of these is sufficient to guarantee good coping. They are, however, prerequisites for whatever is planned or done about psychosocial and personal problems.

Every cancer patient has a story to tell. Few get a chance to tell it. Every physician or nurse has many stories to tell. Few such stories illuminate the principles that guide or demonstrate how best to cope with cancer and its afflicted patients.[5] A collection of stories, an anthology of anecdotes, and a clutch of case reports should be supplemented by rigorous efforts to obtain reliable information from structured interviews, psychological tests, and statistical procedures with as many cancer patients as possible.

Behind every hospital chart of any cancer patient is someone struggling to cope with the immediate impact and prospective problems related to a specific disease and a nonspecific set of remedies. These treatments sometimes cure, but more often simply control for varying lengths of time. Hospital charts seldom clarify the personal plight of cancer patients. Instead, the patient is often reduced to a carrier of disease, stripped of psychosocial implications. What a cancer patient does or does not do to cope effectively is seldom noted and even less often understood.

Cancer, like war, is too serious to be left to the physicians. A cancer patient is more than a vessel for a neoplastic process. Jobs are lost, never regained. Families are split, or draw closer together. Close relationships disintegrate; friendships falter. Conflicts may be aggravated. Values can be sullied. Goals are given up for the pursuit of a cure that may never come. Even new diseases arise as a result of treatment.

I am tempted to minimize, not exaggerate, these extremes, but I am also very sure that cancer cannot be confined to biological boundaries, without human implications. In any event, it can hardly be disputed that medicine needs to know more about what cancer patients who cope well manage to do, and what those who fail do not do.

Which coping strategies are most effective most of the time? How is it that some cancer patients, with about the same amount of disease, are more disabled than others? And even if their survival is approximately equal, what factors and forces influence the course and quality of life?

What is it about a cancer patient that distinguishes him or her from patients with other chronic illnesses? For that matter, what is cancer? According to official publications, over 100 diseases are now covered by the term "cancer."[6] Most of these neoplasms are rare. Although almost any organ can be the site, only a comparatively few major sites involve large enough numbers of patients to make simultaneous and significant psychosocial observations along with physical data.

In order to study psychosocial factors, other features need to be kept relatively constant. These include the site, type of cancer, microscopic appearance, stage of development and differentiation, manner of spread, type of treatment, and so forth. Demographic data are also required, such as age, sex, marital status, ethnic origin, socioeconomic status, siblings, family history, occupation, living conditions, and so on. Only when these objective elements are known, can we understand exactly what cancer patients have as problems and resources.

The lot of a psychosocial investigator is not an easy one. Naturalistic studies of personality and behavior within a psychobiological spectrum are very elusive and ambiguous. The investigator must compromise between *generality, specificity,* and *relevance.*[7] While seeking principles, we are also concerned with the real world of actual people. Generality, specificity, and relevance are not mutually exclusive, but each one is a check on the others, helping to prevent excesses of enthusiasm or bias about any special viewpoint.

The most significant psychosocial variables may be those which are most difficult to detect, define, and measure. In contrast, what is measured most easily may be trivial or irrelevant. For example, it is likely that self-esteem is closely related to how well anyone copes. But how does one define self-esteem clearly enough so that others will understand, verify, or refute? It is much more difficult to define such concepts than, say, to measure height or weight, or to know the birth dates of near relatives.

What are the forces influencing cancer patients? They are not clinical robots who can be kept in isolation, studied only by laboratory tests. Patients are always being bombarded with influences, social and environmental, which can scarcely be enumerated. I am not recounting the tribulations of a psychosocial investigator in order to get sympathy for a complex task. I do so only to emphasize that even the most obvious, uncontroversial generalization can only be true for some people, not everyone. Nevertheless, no one is so unique that his or her characteristics cannot be found in someone else. Moreover, in order to communicate with clarity, it is necessary and permissible to make unqualified generalizations at times, provided that they are based on at least semisolid data. In short, coping can be studied—what it means, how it works, what can be done to strengthen it.

A PATIENT TALKS TO DOCTORS

Busy doctors do not always have the time, interest, or skill to listen well, elicit relevant information, and respond correctly and compassionately. This somewhat paraphrased excerpt from a tumor conference at a well-known hospital may be typical of what many more patients would like to say, had they an opportunity:

> I am a patient who has lived with active cancer for over two years. I have been through the available treatment. Now I know that my chances of living out my life span are not great. . . .
>
> Almost all of you will have a member of your family, close friend, relative, or maybe even yourself develop cancer. All of you have patients like me

who aren't going to be cured by early diagnosis, surgery, radiation, chemotherapy, or anything else.

My surgeon cared a great deal about me, more than I can convey, or will have time to say. But having lived with the disease for so long, I've concluded that some doctors have bigger hangups about cancer than their patients.

Many, maybe most patients adjust eventually . . . know that they have cancer . . . but many doctors still act as if they were an executioner, as if they were to blame.

What I want to impress on you is not about curing or not curing cancer. It is that *every day is precious!* It is precious whether I live two years or twenty. I am managing, and don't need pity or your guilt.

I was frightened, tearful, and absolutely immobilized before my operation. I didn't even know what to ask. I only knew that cancer seems to run in my family, and regardless of how optimistic doctors were at the beginning, it was a bad disease. I was afraid of death, and my chief feeling was one of *overburdening mortality.*

I asked the resident straight out. What could I expect in the long run, short run, and for the next few weeks? Busy as he was, he sat down, and very gently told me the truth as he knew it. I felt much, much better, just knowing something. It was better than being alone with my fears.

Doctors: When you tell a patient not to worry, that is ridiculous—unless it is followed by a *because.* To me, being told not to worry means that the doctor doesn't want to be bothered. I needed the courage to fight, even knowing that fighting is futile. But I can fight better if the doctor has leveled with me. Believe me, imagination conjured up much more terrifying pictures than anything you might say.

Yes, I've had a recurrence. I'm getting sick from chemotherapy. I know it probably won't do me any good. But if I can get some additional time, who knows? Life is still precious, and time is pretty relative. I don't expect a cure, but I need all the help I can get. Don't give up on me or anyone else. Maybe your patients will be the ones to benefit when that wonderful day comes and cancer can be cured.[8]

This woman says it all, especially about what to do until that wonderful day comes and this book is unnecessary. I know nothing more about her. But I thank her and her doctor, just as I do when anyone teaches us that being alive means something, and probably something different to everyone. For her, coping well meant dealing with overburdening mortality. That mortality, of course, is our common allotment. Consequently, telling someone not to worry is hypocritical. Empty reassurance is a hoax. However, she does talk as if all cancer patients have similar feelings just because they share a common predicament.

Note that she cares about her surgeon's caring, long after cure is out of the question. Evidently, he cares enough, too. Otherwise, she would not have appeared at the conference and been permitted to speak at great length (I abbreviated the text). Ordinarily, at tumor conferences, patients are wheeled in and out with monotonous and impersonal regularity. They are sometimes asked a question or two, but hardly given a chance to answer. I often wish I had the temerity to cry out, "Look, we *care* about you!"

Her strategy for coping is confrontation. She wanted more information, got it, then acted accordingly, with much less distress and fear. She is realistically hopeful, not for cure, but for something additional. I suspect that her phrase "Life is precious" is an expression of wholehearted morale in action: to live as long and as well as possible. She recommends that physicians should disavow guilt. It is usually not their fault when a patient is mortally ill.

Obviously, this woman did not need psychiatric consultation, but her problems went beyond the limited scope of the tumor itself. It offended her existence. What would have happened, had she not been so articulate? She did know whom to ask, not what to ask. But suppose she had kept silent? Would anyone have sought or elicited her predominant concerns?

A SURVIVOR TALKS ABOUT DOCTORS

In contrast to the first patient, I quote from a letter sent by a woman hundreds of miles away.

> Dear Dr. Weisman:
>
> I saw an article in the paper about your recent talk. Much of what you said hit home. So I sat down to write, knowing that you'd probably understand. . . . Anyway, I don't have people who care very much. . . .
>
> About 5 years ago, my husband, then 45, died of kidney cancer. The impressions, however, are still so vivid that it could all have happened just this year. . . . His family pretended that he wasn't dying, then they ignored us completely, me and our 9-year-old son.
>
> The most unbelievable thing of all was the attitude of my husband's doctor. He is a very prominent specialist. But he treated my husband for almost 3 years without taking a full history. I don't know why. . . . But for about 8 months before surgery, my husband's kidney hadn't functioned [sic]. He was never checked for cancer, just shuttled in and out so quickly. We trusted the doctor because of his fine reputation. When he decided to operate, we went along.
>
> My husband didn't improve after surgery. The doctor *never* told him that he hadn't removed the kidney because of a tumor, or that he wasn't going to get better. One day I worked up enough courage to ask him to talk things over with my husband. He was pretty busy, and as brusque as ever. "These people instinctively know what's wrong. They don't have to be told." Dr. Weisman, that is bullshit of the worst kind. He was talking about my husband, not "these people." *We needed to know and trust someone.*
>
> As I look back, the most degrading thing was the desertion. Only our minister seemed to care a little, but it helped a lot. Everyone else just came and

went, telling him how great he looked! As the end, only my son and I were around.

Maybe I should have had psychiatric help at some time, but after all, I wasn't insane, and certainly am not now. I'm just a 50-year-old widow with a 15-year-old son who hardly remembers his father. There is still an invisible wall between me and the people who wouldn't share a little bit with us. Man's inhumanity to man is worse than the cancer.

I hope I've given you a broader picture than just one more complaining widow. I can still hear the floor nurse saying to me, "If he deteriorates, he can stay here. If not, there's nothing more to do, and he'll have to go."

There was so much to be done, and we needed so little.

Sincerely,

(name omitted by me)

This letter is as eloquent as the comments of the patient who spoke at the conference. Five years after her husband's death, she was still aggrieved enough to reach out to someone she had only read about. Perhaps there was nothing more to do, but she might have received help at an earlier time when she and her husband were helplessly awaiting death by themselves. So little was needed.

The best time to offer support and to assess distress is at the start of illness, not years later, nor even when death is at the threshold. Of course, some patients will not accept or need specific help earlier, but an evaluation can still be done.

The floor nurse offered the customary paradox: "He can stay only if he promises to get worse and die without being too long about it!" Glaser and Strauss documented the perils of a dying patient who takes too long.[9] The staff gets frustrated and angry, often quite unwittingly.

Once again, psychiatric consultation was unnecessary and might even have been refused. Counseling would have been wholly acceptable, although some cancer patients deem it a test of strength to "make it on my own," as if counselors would have it otherwise. Social service is not mentioned. Perhaps the few social workers in this very small town were already overburdened with the machinery of nursing home placement and money matters of other patients who were even worse off.

A VERY BAD DEATH

Registries, statistics, and year-end reports usually offer very little information that a psychosocial investigator can use. Socioeconomic status, occupation, family size, church attendance, and other elementary social data from which one might infer a great deal are simply not recorded.[10] Consequently, unless special efforts are made, correlations of cancer with psychosocial factors depend on analyzing individual case reports.

Even though the public at large may believe that death is always an unmitigated evil, this is but one of many misconceptions about death.[11] Some deaths *are* better than others. Despite adequate medical treatment, attentive social service, and other more intangible factors, beneficial or detrimental, the following patient died a very bad death, with much distress and inadequate coping.

Case 1

During his 46 years, Tony was rarely ill. He worked hard in a factory, and managed to support a family of eight. But one day, after losing about 10 pounds over several weeks and coughing blood periodically, he came to the clinic. He was found to have oat cell carcinoma of the lung, with metastases to regional lymph nodes and to the liver. The only treatment was palliative chemotherapy.

Marie, his wife, insisted that Tony not be told anything. "It would kill him!" Therefore, nothing was said until about 3 months later. Then, almost off hand, Tony asked a clinic doctor about his progress. Very gently, the doctor told him about the tumor, but was very optimistic about the long-range prospect of recovery. After this brief talk, Tony felt less distressed. He complained very little and needed fewer opiates for pain. Most of the time, however, before and after the exchange with the doctor, Tony bickered incessantly with his wife and children. He talked about going back to work, even though the factory had not been in contact with him.

Officially, Tony was unaware of the gloomy prognosis. Nevertheless, during one of several hospitalizations, he had two revealing dreams: (1) He was moved from a large, pleasant hospital room to a dark and lonely cubicle. He called out, but no one answered. He was completely alone. (2) He and a favorite daughter were on a space ship, headed somewhere out in infinity. He knew that this was a one-way trip, and they would never return.

Although Tony talked about work, he had no job and was hardly able to move around their small quarters. The family was broke and had to accept public welfare. He asked no questions about finances. His brothers and sisters offered nothing. He complained of chest pain, insomnia, cough, and progressive weight loss. Because he had never been sick until he came to the hospital, he rationalized that the treatment caused all his troubles. "If I don't get any more treatment, I should be feeling better soon." No further treatment was planned. Tony did voice fewer complaints, because he became too weak to complain.

He remained almost immobilized in a constant state of resentment and pain. Once in a while, he talked about being afraid to die. He spoke about his father and sister, who also died of cancer, and with whom he expected to be reunited. Later, Marie reported that Tony slept with a picture of his dead father by his side. He was also troubled about leaving her with a double burden of being without funds, and having a problem with their son, who was a drug addict. He openly wondered about killing his son, who was once a favorite. This would not only relieve Marie, but "no one would send a dying man to jail." He resented the hospital because after so much treatment, he was worse than ever. Marie resented religion; she had prayed at first for his recovery, but the answer had been to live at a terrible price in suffering. Gradually, Tony refused to eat or speak. He resisted nursing care and medication. Finally, he was transferred to a terminal care facility, where he died one day later.

What went wrong? Doctors had been reasonably supportive, I suppose. They drew off pleural fluid regularly, and provided him with ample opiates. Yet the family interpreted these efforts as unnecessary and even harmful. The hospital was to blame, they reasoned. Tony and Marie fought vociferously, as long as possible, before settling into more subdued embitterment. Months later, of course, she idealized their relationship, admiring the stoicism with which he faced death. His fellow workers did not help, or even show interest. He and his late father both worked in the same factory for many years and were simply cut off the payroll when they became ill.

One cannot underestimate the injury and humiliation inflicted by unemployment, welfare, and witnessing one's transition from a sturdy, somewhat self-sufficient breadwinner to a helpless invalid, awaiting death. The problem of having a son destined for another kind of death also seemed like an extra burden. His son, too, would be better off dead.

What else might have been done? More open discussions intended to face reality without rancor? Enlisting some tangible appreciation from the factory for long years of service? Foster home care for the smaller children? Talking with Tony's brothers and sisters about providing more for this family? Looking back, perhaps not much could have been changed. But other families who are, seemingly, no less impoverished gather together and come to terms with the inevitable, without fallacious resentment. Should a similar situation occur again, as it must, our cue will be to muster every available resource, as the inexorable decline develops.

A VERY GOOD DEATH

Most of us cherish an illusion that anticipates a healthy and secure old age, steeped in dignity, wisdom, and productive leisure. Death, if contemplated at all, is postponed to an indefinite future, like a receding horizon that one never quite reaches. A good death, therefore, is the next best thing to not dying at all. It is but an extension of a good life, in which there is only long survival, no sickness or economic concerns, abiding emotional support, and high self-regard. Fortunately, however, only because good deaths do not require ideal conditions, a very good death is within reach of many people.

Case 2

Phillip had been a successful banker, married for over 45 years, and father of three children, who kept in close contact with their parents, although living far apart.

Since his retirement at 66, Phillip led essentially the same life as before. He worked part-time, read, attended church, and participated in community activities. He enjoyed golf, smoking, investing in the market, and visiting with friends. His retirement reflected good planning and a good life. He achieved success through his own efforts, had strong family ties, and a happy marriage, without significant conflict. His abiding fear, however, was that he might live too long and become senile, as happened to his father.

One day, shortly after his 68th birthday, Phillip consulted the family doctor. For over a year he felt unusually fatigued, lost a little weight, and seemed less interested in events than customary. The physician referred Phillip to an eminent surgeon after taking a chest x-ray. A small adenocarcinoma in the right lung was resected. Phillip was completely informed about the lesion, including the favorable prognosis.

In the months that followed, Phillip never regained the zest he once knew. Outwardly, his life was unchanged. Inside, much was different. He faced mortality candidly, however, because he now knew that, regardless of longevity, it was unlikely that he would live long enough to become senile. He was glad when each day was over; fatigue was mounting, even with moderate activity.

Phillip realized when progress ceased and his weariness grew. Nine months after the operation, a chest x-ray showed that now both lungs were affected. He accepted chemotherapy, but knew that the outcome would not significantly be affected. Nevertheless, he remained quietly optimistic, somewhat stoical, and, as far as possible, self-reliant. Little by little, he became confined to home and church, with an occasional trip to his office. He had few complaints, aside from awkwardness and ataxia brought on by chemotherapy.

One Sunday, two of his children arrived for a visit. For the first time, Phillip suggested that the family go on to church without him, because he was just too tired. On the way, his wife suddenly thought that this might be Phillip's last day. This, too, was strange because she had been much more optimistic than he, hoping for a long reprieve. As if by prearrangement, when they returned from church, Phillip was sitting in his favorite chair, dead.

The contrast between Tony and Phillip could hardly be more extreme. Their lives were as different as their deaths. But age, money, and social status are not the only ways in which Tony and Phillip differed. Tony had much pain. Phillip was simply fatigued. Tony had many family problems, including a drug addict son who threatened to remain a troublesome antisocial individual. Phillip's family was unwavering in their loyalty, despite distance. Tony argued incessantly with his wife, who wanted to "protect" him from the supposedly noxious effect of knowing about the diagnosis. Phillip's wife quietly shared information about his cancer. Their relationship was calm, respectful, and supportive. Tony seemed to know little about the cancer, aside from what a physician told him on one occasion. His dreams and behavior disclosed, however, that he knew much more, and expected to join his father and sister after death. Phillip was not only kept informed, but even anticipated the decline before his own doctor knew that cancer had spread. Tony was bitter; Phillip was resigned. Phillip preferred to die before becoming senile. In a sense, he chose to die when he did. Tony resisted and resented any intrusion, blaming the hospital for making him sick. Phillip attracted friends, while Tony had no friends, even after working at the same factory for many years.

HOPE, TRUST, AND THE QUALITY OF SURVIVAL

The difference between a very bad death and a very good death cannot be ascribed simply to having more symptoms and less money. Obviously, pain is more difficult to tolerate than fatigue. But social status implies other kinds of assets, even though both men had cancer of the lung.

Phillip's higher socioeconomic status allowed him certain privileges that Tony's marginal life did not. There were undoubtedly differences in intelligence, domestic relationships, and social support systems. Because so many factors and forces must be considered when assessing any patient's potential for a good life, or, for that matter, a good death, three major categories of information are used: *disease* (diagnosis, site, stage, symptoms, treatment, comorbidity, and so forth), *personality* (character traits, optimism, intelligence, interests, previous successes and failure, and so on), and *social context* (key relationships, work, finances, religion, family).

There are many patients with ample financial resources who are impoverished in other respects. But people from lower socioeconomic strata have a hard time anyway, and the way in which cancer disrupts their life is no exception. Patients who are accustomed to success see to it that they get good medical care, and that the people they trust are trustworthy.

There is no doubt that, in general, patients who are well off have it better. But these factors, like medical symptoms, do not guarantee a good survival. For example, successful excision of a malignant melanoma may be a happy and conclusive event. Sometimes, however, the result is good only from the surgeon's viewpoint. For the patient, a "good" medical result is an unsightly scar that prevents social activity, undermines self-confidence, and presents itself as a memento of a constant worry. In contrast, some patients with bowel cancer and regional metastases are still able to work and function much as before, despite their colostomy.

Good coping, regardless of the medical outcome, is clearly an extension of how well a patient coped during healthier days. However, part of coping well depends on the social context, including supportive others. Here, too, one finds difficulties, because the social context is also a social contract: one is acceptable, provided that ordinary functions and social roles are preserved. This means that disease or even a history of a serious illness is kept hidden. Consequently, some cancer patients continue working, regardless of how sick they feel inside. They know that cancer frightens people, and that the cancer patient symbolizes such fears. Nothing, therefore, is said. As a result, there are patients who do not complain, and do well, seemingly, until a few days before death. They are not especially stoical, but wish fervently for privacy, as if significant others can tolerate only so much. Thus, trust has its limitations and conditions.

Hope, trust, and the quality of survival are mutually related factors. Whatever damages one impairs the others. False reassurances, exhortations about courage, sermons about strength, and deceptions about the future do not fortify hope, but undermine trust, and ruin the remaining quality of life.

Hope is an intangible, immeasurable, and very real sentiment. It is produced by optimism, expectation, and recollections of past success and failure. According to Stotland, hope is a learned response, augmented by the example of supportive and successful others.[12] Mere words are very transient and generally ineffectual, unless mutual confidence silently conveys itself. Very hopeful people set goals for themselves, and try hard to reach them, trusting others when necessary. It is the determined person who succeeds, not the aggressive. Most cancer patients do not depend on hope alone, nor do they hope exclusively for recovery, extended survival, or return to previous ways of life. Hope is designed to see people through adversity, because it is a character trait, not because it can be strategically generated or discouraged.

When hopeful people acquire cancer, they are tenacious and resourceful. Therefore, hope is not simply a wish to undo what cannot be changed, nor does it evaporate at bad news. Hopeful people, strangely enough, do not depend as much on goals as upon self-concept, even though self-concept is nourished by success in reaching goals.

Confidence in another person, which we call trust, requires mutuality. It cannot be sustained unless both people trust each other. The woman at the tumor conference trusted her physician, who evidently reciprocated. Candor from the surgical resident kept up her morale, but the resident also trusted her. Even with dim expectations about chemotherapy, she maintained hope, feeling that life was precious. Under the circumstances, quality of survival was also good. The woman who wrote me had been deserted. There was no trust. Her morale was broken. She was bitter, and hope was gone. Quality of survival, even after her husband's death, remained low.

Hope is a prerequisite for good coping. There is also counterfeit hope which masquerades as optimism. Genuine hope does not need denial, because good copers seek and use resources of all kinds. Counterfeit hope only pretends to cope. Actually, it covers passivity.

Hope and trust are sturdy enough to withstand truth. True acceptance is based on hope, not for cure, necessarily, but for a good quality of life. Cancer patients must contend with impermanence and uncertainty more than is true for most illnesses. Nevertheless, the four patients I have referred to (the woman at the conference, the husband of the widow who wrote, Tony and his very bad death, Phillip with a very good death) all shared the inevitability of disease. Their differences in plight depended largely on non-physical factors. Whether psychosocial factors can actually extend survival is a matter for further study.[13] But hope, trust, quality of survival, and reasonable control of symptoms are principal parts of that action called "coping well."

REFERENCES

1 Evans, J., *Living with a Man Who Is Dying,* Taplinger Publishing Co. Inc., New York, 1971.
2 Bell, T., *In the Midst of Life,* Atheneum Publishers, New York, 1961.
3 Gibson, W., *A Mass for the Dead,* Atheneum Publishers, New York, 1968.
4 Alsop, S., *Stay of Execution: A Sort of Memoir,* J. B. Lippincott Company, Philadelphia, 1973.
5 Abrams, R., *Not Alone with Cancer: A Guide for Those Who Care,* Charles C Thomas, Springfield, Ill., 1974.
6 " '75 Cancer Facts & Figures," American Cancer Society.
7 Weisman, A., "Suicide, Death and Life-threatening Behavior," in H. Resnick and B. Hathorne (eds.), *Suicide Prevention in the Seventies,* National Institute of Mental Health, Department of Health, Education and Welfare Publication 72-9054, Washington, 1973, chap. III, pp. 13–18.
8 "Every Day Is Precious," *CA—A Cancer Journal for Clinicians,* **22**:1, 70–72, January/February 1972.
9 Glaser, B., and A. Strauss, *Time for Dying,* Aldine Publishing Company, Chicago, 1968.
10 Silverberg, E., "Cancer Statistics, 1977," *CA—A Cancer Journal for Clinicians,* **27**:1, 26–41, January/February 1977.
11 Weisman, Avery D., "Misgivings and Misconceptions in the Psychiatric Care of Terminal Patients," *Psychiatry,* **33**:1, 67–81, February 1970.
12 Stotland, E., *The Psychology of Hope,* Jossey-Bass, Inc., Publishers, San Francisco, 1969.
13 Worden, J. W., L. C. Johnston, and R. H. Harrison, "Survival Quotient as a Method for Investigating Psychosocial Aspects of Cancer Survival," *Psychological Reports,* **35**:719–726, 1974.

Safe Conduct

The existential event of cancer cannot be walled off from the rest of one's life. Like the illness, it can insidiously spread, even if carefully monitored. The four patients I chose in illustrating critical issues about coping and getting help with coping all had fatal outcomes. This was not designed to frighten anyone, nor was it deliberately grim. The possibility of death from cancer is a reality that must be confronted before one can intelligently comprehend the full meaning of coping with cancer. Fear of death is practically universal, but like many other phobias, it can be dissipated by resolute counteraction and confrontation, coupled with an appreciation of how many other factors contribute to that fear, besides the fact of death.[1]

Cancer can be cured, or at least so goes the slogan. It would, however, be a disservice to imply that there is really nothing much to worry about, and that an absolute cure for all kinds of cancer will be here before the ink is dry on this page.

Meanwhile, the fact that so many cancer patients cope very well is an encouraging indication that the ramifications of having cancer can be contained. Good coping starts with the patient and with trust in those whom that patient turns to. Safe conduct is, for the physician, an obligation, duty, and an indispensable quality in successfully managing a treacherous situation.

A world that flings disaster about so indiscriminately needs all the confrontation and coping we can muster, just to contend with primitive fears that abound in us all. Coping requires recognition that a problem exists, then doing something about it. Good coping means (1) good solutions for old problems, (2) adequate solutions for new problems, and (3) resourceful solutions for unexpected problems. There is coping for short-term and for long-term problems, which are often not the same. Avoidance has limited use.

No less an authority than Hippocrates gave cancer its name. This dubious tribute drew upon the analogy of a crab that creeps along quietly with claws that reach out in all directions. The name probably also had some relation to the lore of astrology. I mention this because the very term "cancer" evokes ancient fears and superstitions. None of us is wholly immune to belief in magic, fatalism, and meaningless rituals, sanctioned by long practice.

LAGTIME

The first concern of newly diagnosed cancer patients and their family or friends is about life and death. This must be faced and talked about, without attempting to prophesize. Just to recognize a prevalent concern is enough to begin with, before going on to coping proper. Recognition of a fear, such as the uncertainty facing a new cancer patient, is the basis of good coping through confrontation. The fact that the proportion of total cancer cases who will be saved is steadily increasing is a happy thought, but not really relevant to the individual. However, prediagnostic coping with awareness that something is wrong may itself be a clue to how that individual will cope with future distress. Therefore, many reasons can be found for delay.

Lapse of time between early symptoms and later diagnosis is not a sure indicator of negligence or denial. What is out of sight is easy to put out of mind. Delay, or, more precisely, "lagtime," can be a sign of fearful procrastination or a trait of independent self-reliance. A 58-year-old woman noticed a lump in her breast for about two years before consulting a physician, when the lesion started to bleed. She offered no excuses, aside from the conventional "I thought it would go away." Inquiry disclosed, however, that she was deserted by her husband many years earlier. She worked as a waitress and domestic in order to support five children. She was proud of her record, children, and of "keeping troubles to myself and not asking for help." Her sister had already died of breast cancer. But the strategies of self-reliance and "keep troubles inside and don't ask for help" prevented her from getting medical help earlier.

Delay is not necessarily due to indifference or fear of what a doctor might find.[2] But patients usually find ready reasons to procrastinate. "I wanted to wait until after my daughter's wedding," "Why borrow trouble?" "This is my busy season." As long as uncertainty exists, some people wait and wait, while others rush to consult a physician in order to relieve anxiety. Prompt action is not always a sign of prudence, nor is delay, deplorable. Overt denial, however, in the presence, say, of an erosive lesion of the face is, fortunately, quite rare. More common is the patient who knows from some inner perception that cancer might be present, but manages to put off the definite diagnosis by a physician. Unlike the patient who kept troubles to herself, long lagtime is not often a testimony to courage in facing adversity. One woman had an encrusted lesion of her breast for over 10 years. The cancer would not have been discovered, had she not developed intestinal obstruction from a second tumor, this time affecting the colon.

Somewhere between the very prompt and the procrastinating patient are people who seek checkups just to make sure nothing is wrong, even though years may have elapsed since their previous examination. In fact, most cancer patients delay no longer than about 8 weeks after the initial symptoms appear, regardless of the site.[3] Naturally, a tumor that causes obstruction or bleeding reduces lagtime, while a tumor without specific symptoms is tolerated longer.

Reasons for postponing an examination are as complicated as human nature itself. Physicians are no exception in seeking excuses and rationalizations to avoid a showdown.[4] Fatalism and superstition sometimes cause people to believe that nothing can be done, anyway, so why bother? They confuse the diagnosis of cancer with terminal illness, which is, of course, an incorrect assumption. However, prediagnostic pessimism often reflects a general attitude toward other problems: apathetic surrender, resistance is impossible, fate will have its way.

There are also people who firmly believe that virtue is rewarded, and that being "good," i.e., abstemious, conscientious, prudent, and pious, will protect them. One man said, "I kept such a clean house, better than any woman. I was afraid that if I got married, my wife would dirty up the place." So he kept a clean house, obeyed all rules, avoided risks, and died of cancer, just as he might have succumbed to anything else, including accident or another disease. But he was convinced that cancer is a dirty disease, not neat and clean, like a heart attack. Unfortunately, this is a common prejudice.

INFORMED UNCERTAINTY

Uncertainty is difficult to tolerate at any time. Either through ignorance or misguided compassion, physicians may tacitly contribute to delay by bland reassurance, curt dismissal, or negligence. "Come back to see me in six months. If it's not gone, we'll check into it."

The aims of medicine are (1) to prevent unnecessary deaths, (2) to help patients live as long and well as possible, and (3) to circumvent the human obligation to die. These are often confused, tragically at times. The first aim, preventing unnecessary deaths or restoring people to health, is usually quite feasible. The second aim, helping people live longer and better lives, is more difficult and uncertain. The third aim, circumventing death indefinitely, is impossible.

Every patient has a right to accurate diagnosis, prompt treatment, adequate relief, and safe conduct. Problems of *accurate diagnosis* belong to textbooks of medicine. But some patients call up for a routine physical examination, and deliberately conceal their concern about a worrisome symptom. Then they leave reassured that if anything had been wrong, the doctor would have discovered it. Routine reasons are frequently no reasons at all. The physician is therefore wise to ask why any patient seeks examination at a particular time. "What prompted you to ask for a routine physical examination *just now?*"

Prompt treatment is a right that follows accurate diagnosis. It does not mean premature treatment for an illness that may not exist. Prompt treatment or referral for it is intended to prevent unnecessary delay, when enough information is available or could be obtained by appropriate tests. Regardless of motives, the doctor who inordinately delays, waffles, and misses the diagnosis will always be blamed. Short-term reassurance may make a nervous patient feel good, but it can lead to long-term regrets and resentments. Fine differences in phraseology are forgotten; gallantry is unimportant; distortion and maximization of small differences are the rule, especially in retrospect. "My doctor must have thought I was neurotic or something. He kept telling me to come back in 3 months, and not to worry. I didn't want to trouble him, so I never called back at all." Recall that the woman at the conference cautioned doctors never to say, "Don't worry," unless it was followed by "Because. . . . " Some physicians have a way of skimming over the fine print of inherent uncertainty when they tell a newly postoperative cancer patient, "Well, we got it all!" They really mean "We got as much out as possible; there may be more." Patients are usually so relieved that they hesitate to ask the next logical question, "What exactly does 'getting it all' mean?" If the doctor truly believes that no further risk is involved, she can say so. If, however, further treatment is indicated, she can also admit uncertainty, without losing optimism or alarming the patient.

Few patients accuse their physician of being an alarmist. On the contrary, patients are pleased with being taken seriously. Though they may grumble about expenses, thoroughness is appreciated. "The doctor said it might be nothing, but he wanted to be sure." "I hate to be a complainer, but Dr. X said I was right in coming to him when I did."

The third aim, *adequate relief,* is an adjunct to prompt treatment. It is designed to help nature cure its own, not to hide the diagnosis. For example, family medicine is now a rapidly growing specialty, far from the general practitioner of a generation or two ago.[5] It has thrived on better definition of a primary physician's comprehensive role in a complex society. This means, briefly, to understand that patients and families are social units that interact, thus aggravating physical illnesses or simulating physical illnesses because of psychosocial tensions. Adequate relief, therefore, is not just prescribing painkillers, soporifics, or practicing palliative medicine. It is the result of alert, diversified, and ingenious intercessions.

Pain, local symptoms, and systemic complaints are found in many cases of cancer, as well as in other maladies. Systemic complaints are, by definition, hard to describe, define, and even more difficult to diagnose. Weight loss, insomnia, weakness, fatigue, and so forth are often considered "psychosomatic," and therefore "entitled" to be ignored. Many dimensions of illness need to be considered. No instrumentality can be ignored when it comes to relieving distress. The schism between mental, emotional, and physical is an artifact. "I feel very tired all the time," may mean anemia. But it can also mean, "I feel very tired all the time. . . . I can't work, so I am getting discouraged as each day passes, wondering if I'll ever get better." Long drawn-out fatigue can mask many illnesses, and sometimes prompts a patient to make a self-diagnosis of exclusion, namely, not calling a doctor's attention to a new lump, a swollen gland, or a change in bowel habits.

SAFE CONDUCT

Safe conduct is that dimension beyond diagnosis, treatment, and relief which refers to how a physician will conduct a patient through a maze of uncertain, perplexing, and distressing events. It means to behave prudently while guiding a patient, such as one with cancer, through the perilous unknown. It does not mean that the doctor is punctiliously correct according to a script of convention, caution, and rigid routine. Good behavior is taken for granted.

Safe conduct should not be confused with rehabilitation or psychotherapy. These are subspecialties of experts who see comparatively few cancer patients. While a primary physician cannot reduce all danger and distress, he or she can be constantly cool, courteous, forbearing, and courageous.

The latter is not a universal trait. Doctors can wince or be apprehensive themselves. It takes more than intellectual integrity to say, "I don't know, but we'll try to find out." Some doctors prefer treating patients who will certainly get well, bother them very little, but be deeply appreciative. Safe conduct is scarcely an issue in these cases. For a cancer patient, however, safe conduct is assured when the doctor is accessible, not at all times, but at times of need. Accessibility can relieve anguish and make uncertainty tolerable. I find it baffling, and so must patients, that a patient can be in the hospital for days or weeks, without even knowing the names of primary physicians or nurses. To some extent, this is a way of life for patients from lower socioeconomic stations, but good treatment does not mean treatment by a committee of anonymous technicians. In short, there is no safe conduct without individualization.

WHAT TO DO ABOUT TRUTH

Truth is not easy to deal with. Otherwise, so many people, including physicians, would not shade truth or delegate it to someone else. All tests have, let us say, been completed, including biopsy, x-ray, and so forth. Good coping requires that a patient have sufficient information to participate in decisions. An informed patient, as I shall repeat from time to time, is a better patient. But truth is a process, not a circumscribed body of unequivocal facts that never change. Its contribution to coping is that doctor and patient now share a common reality. At this point, my emphasis is on the physician, because he or she is usually charged with the responsibility of telling the truth and explaining otherwise mystifying procedures. When patients turn to others, it is to circumvent the physician, as if they are afraid of being misled, deceived, or even of being told the "truth."

The most frequent question asked about a newly diagnosed cancer patient is whether or not to tell the truth. Families may demand silence, deception, or conspiracy to shield their relative. "Don't tell him. He'll just give up." "If she knew the truth, she'd fall apart and commit suicide." "He's never been very stable, and he couldn't take it." This response is understandable, but mistaken.

Here, statistics may be revealing. According to various surveys, physicians are reluctant to tell cancer patients the diagnosis, even if by so doing, no harm would befall the patient.[6] On the other hand, most lay persons surveyed declare that they would want to know their diagnosis, under all circumstances.[7] Our findings show that only about 10 percent of newly diagnosed cancer patients are somewhat guarded about the facts of their illness, and feel that they already know enough to permit treatment. They willingly depend upon the doctor's discretion for further information. The rest want the "truth."

There is a difference between knowing the truth and knowing how much can be appropriately used.[8] A shut-off point beyond which one can only conjecture is a matter of individual judgment. Modern emphasis on informed consent, human studies, and individual responsibility makes it imperative that any cancer patient be familiar with major information about illness and proposed treatment. The old-time presumption that doctor always knows best, and that the best patients ask no questions and therefore know as little as possible is as obsolete as writing prescriptions in illegible Latin. Nevertheless, some physicians discourage questions or are unavailable, especially if questions are repetitive. But every patient has a right to basic information, as well as a right to refuse a recounting of unwelcome details.

When families insist on secrecy, however, physicians ought not to accede automatically. Families usually do this out of their own anguish, not from malice or will to deceive. As a rule, asking for deception reflects a poor relationship within the family. Suicide is extremely rare among cancer patients, especially as a result of learning the diagnosis (see Chapter 5). Nevertheless, this is a hoary excuse offered by apprehensive doctors and fearful families, as if bearers of bad tidings were to blame or that truth by itself could kill. Secrecy does no one any service. It bars effective communication and stalls coping. Moreover, an adult may feel abandoned, alone, baffled, apprehensive, as well as, justifiably, insulted by being left out. Desertion at moments of truth creates a distance that may be more devastating than the diagnosis. Distress is largely determined by *how* a patient is told about cancer, not *what* he or she is told.

Most patients suspect the diagnosis, anyway. At least, they infer a great deal from silence and uncharacteristic behavior. That is not to say that "these people" know without being told. Such "groupthink" betrays safe conduct and communication, and undermines future coping.

Defenses against the diagnosis, however, are not infrequent. Patients refrain from voicing suspicion for three main reasons: (1) to allow a loophole, (2) to gain time, and (3) to protect someone. One woman allowed herself a loophole by saying that while her surgeon discussed the operation in considerable detail, he hadn't mentioned the diagnosis. Officially, she knew nothing about "cancer." She merely surmised that he had reasons for not talking about what she already suspected. Another patient exclaimed suddenly, "Everyone seems to know about my illness, but me!" A third woman patient curtly said, "I don't know what's wrong, and I'm not ready to!" The last comment gains time, assuming that the less said, the better, and what one doesn't know may not be true.

Protecting others is a common tactic. One woman even gave her physician optimistic but incorrect reports when he visited on morning rounds.

Because she really felt quite ill, I asked what her doctor said that day. "Oh, I haven't told him. He has tried so hard; my family has been through so much. I don't want to disappoint them."

HOW TO TELL

I find something a little pathetic about this exchange:

DR.:   No, I haven't told him about the diagnosis, and he hasn't asked.
ADW: I wonder why he hasn't asked.
DR.:   I think he knows anyway.
ADW: Then why not talk about it? He certainly must have some questions.
DR.:   I doubt it. Otherwise, he'd ask. These people somehow know without being told.
ADW: Which people?

And so the conversation might go on, with more and more circularity and rationalization. Sometimes, a psychiatrist, nurse, or social worker is caught in a crossfire of distortion, despite being very circumspect about transgressing upon professional prerogatives.

It is not amiss for the doctor to initiate discussion, mustering enough courage to say, "Mr. A, you haven't asked me anything about your illness and what treatment I've planned. Perhaps something holds you back."

When telling a patient about cancer is too perfunctory or routine, the doctor has become callous. When it is too difficult, the doctor has too much anxiety, and needs to recognize his or her own guilt or anxiety. Equivocation is apt to lead to confusion, not clarity. Statistics about what percentage of patients do this or that provide useful background information, but it is hardly a basis for individual prognosis. Informed uncertainty, however, is tolerable, besides being more accurate and even more specific. Physicians are sometimes tempted to engage patients and families in differential diagnosis, as if they were colleagues or medical students ("It could be this, it might be that, but I don't think so"). These are delaying, defusing tactics, not far removed from telling encouraging anecdotes about knowing someone who. . . .

The ideal strategy is *candor with hope.* Tact, compassion, common sense, and straightforward statements are safeguards against platitudes, circumlocutions, apologetics, and inane irrelevancies. Euphemisms do have a place, particularly if the very word "cancer" is likely to stir up too many emotions. Technical distinctions can also be valuable, but this is different from pseudoscientific claptrap and mystification. "The doctor said that the tumor was just about to turn malignant." "She said it was more like chronic infection that takes a lot more time to get rid of." Half-lies help no one.

One of the important principles of how to tell is to know the difference between uttering words and using language well. When communication is comfortable, language is simple, acceptance increases, distress is minimal, and endless discussion about remote implications of having cancer is unnecessary.

Strategies for telling a cancer patient about the diagnosis and initial treatment are only prototypes for future communication. There are three main tactics, called "hard tell," "soft tell," and "no tell." Hard tell limits itself to bare, unadorned, unqualified facts. It reflects a necessary, but nasty job, done with dispatch. Soft tell is tactful. It allows for shock, bewilderment, closing off, and for patients who only hear half of what is said. No tell is either that or telling an outright lie. "When he's feeling better, I'll tell him," means "When I'm feeling up to it, perhaps I can tell and not tell at the same time."

There are many strategies for not giving information. Almost anyone needs time to assimilate, cogitate, and ask again. The only way to be sure is to inquire about further questions a day or so later, and be prepared to repeat. The following examples are different kinds of communication, terse and tactful, succinct and expansive, with patients who were found to have cancer of the pancreas.

DR.:   Mr. A, we found a bad situation at operation. You have a cancer growing in the pancreas; there is nothing much we can do about it.

DR.:   Mr. B, the cause of your stomach pain is more serious than I hoped. There is a cancer behind your stomach that can't be removed, but we'll try to treat it, anyway.

DR.:   Mr. C, the operation went fine. I expect you'll be feeling better soon. I am sorry that the operation showed a tumor that probably caused your pain and jaundice. I removed as much as I could, and this will help. The tumor is still there, and can't be entirely taken out. It's hard to contain the tumor, but there are other forms of treatment that will be considered. I'll talk more with you about it later on.

DR.:   Mr. D, we did find a tumor. I wish it was possible to clear it up entirely, but it isn't. Other treatment may help. I am sure this news has to be disturbing. I know that I would be, in your place. I don't expect you to be much different from other people. Please let me answer your questions, if I can. I want you to know that I intend to stick by you.

DR.:   Mr. E, the operation went fine. We found the cause of your pain. Other treatments will be coming along, just to make sure. But enough of that for now. See you tomorrow.

In none of these illustrations has the doctor lied. Mr. A got the hard tell. Mr. B's tell was slightly softer, but still somewhat abrupt. Mr. C had the soft tell, and Mr. D was given more information than necessary, including an implication that all was hopeless ("I'll stick by you"). For Mr. E, the doctor used the no tell strategy.

Should a patient ask, "You say I have a tumor. Does that mean cancer?" the doctor must answer. "Yes, you have a form of cancer, but cancer means many things. Some cancers can be treated better than others." If the patient persists, "Is my kind treatable or incurable?" the doctor may be obliged to say, "It is not the kind that responds best to the treatments we have. I do plan, however, to give you chemotherapy or radiation, depending on what our consultants think will be best."

Words may injure, but they do not kill. Similarly, they will not cure, but may vastly ameliorate distress, giving a patient time to reflect, ask questions, or just be silent. Safe conduct requires hope, trust, and compassion for a fellow sufferer. Promise no more than can reasonably be expected or fulfilled. This is the essence of authentic support, not mere reassurance.

THE MORE VULNERABLE PATIENT

Obviously, telling some patients about cancer will be more distressing than telling others. Few cancer patients are so stoical that the news finds them fully prepared and without questions. However, it is not unusual for a patient to close off, nodding numbly, without comprehending the doctor. Others respond as if they had not quite heard. "Oh, I see. Well, now what? I suppose that means everything is O.K., doesn't it?" Some may show a little disbelief. "You weren't sure when I saw you in the office. Can you be absolutely sure now?"

Silence should not be confused with acceptance. Denial and rationalization are not uncommon. "I guess that means I'll have to take it easy for awhile. When can I go back to work?" The impact of cancer has a wide range of responses, not completely determined by physical facts. However, a patient with a localized lesion needing limited treatment is at a psychosocial advantage. At the other extreme, someone with a far-advanced cancer and few psychosocial assets can be expected to cope less effectively and to be more distressed.

Just who *is* the more vulnerable cancer patient? Physical symptoms, advanced staging, and rapid proliferation are, of course, ominous signs. Beyond these dire facts, however, there are patients who are born losers, and expect the future to be no different from the past. Their pessimism may be justified, but they also may have current concerns and past regrets that increase distress. Support from others is minimal, or at best, questionable. Lasting loyalty is simply not there. In fact, people who are confirmed loners cope better than those with shabby support systems, which includes bad marriages.[9]

The least vulnerable cancer patients are those who are optimistic, expecting support from others, and getting it. Communication is always open. If it is not, then such patients demand attention, and will not numbly submit without question. As redundant as it is, resourceful people have ample resources to draw upon. They are usually amiable, but firm and articulate when necessary, and accustomed to success. They may even live longer, with the same disease. If not, the quality of their life will still be better than that of the more marginal person.

Cancer does not confer emotional immunity. Patients with a history of psychiatric problems also tend to be more vulnerable to the emotional complications of cancer.

The diagnosis of emotional vulnerability in newly diagnosed cancer patients is not confined to information about pessimism, marital problems, expected support, and psychiatric treatment. People like to put themselves in the best light, especially when talking with a professional whose respect they want. Consequently, the more vulnerable a cancer patient seems to be, the more difficult it is to get direct confirmation of distress. Notice the difference between the two following approaches.

Wrong:
DR.: Are you a pessimist?
PT.: No, I'm not.
DR.: Do you always look on the gloomy side?
PT.: No, I always look for the best in people.

Right:
DR.: I wonder what happens to you when things you've looked forward to don't turn out right, or you're disappointed.
PT.: Oh, I don't ask for very much, just a little consideration from my family now and then, because I do try hard.
DR.: They don't always appreciate how hard you try. But, as a rule, how do things work out for you in the long run?
PT.: Sometimes things work out, mostly they don't.
DR.: Try as you do, things turn out wrong and you're disappointed. But how do you *ordinarily* expect them to turn out?
PT.: Expect? I'm always surprised when something goes well. I wait for the worst to happen, if you know what I mean. But I'm not what you'd call a pessimist the way some people are. For instance. . . .

HELPING PATIENTS COPE

Safe conduct not only demands that the warning signals of vulnerability be recognized early, but that firm alliances begin and continue throughout the course, regardless of outcome. Physicians should not assume that everyone with cancer will be anxious, depressed, irritable, and so on. Temporary distress is not a reliable sign of persistent future vulnerability. Physical and psychosocial disabilities do tend to meld. "I can't walk by myself" is a report of a physical disability, but it also keeps that patient from working or taking care of a household. "I can't walk and can't work" is a psychosocial problem. The consequence may be, "I can't be like I once was. I am a burden, and no good to anyone."

Helping a vulnerable cancer patient cope better requires help that is optimistic, resourceful, realistic, and so on. If physicians negativistically believe that cancer is a deadly disease, they cannot offer safe conduct. They, too, need help with countercoping (see Chapter 9). The syllogism "Nothing can be done for cancer—this is a cancer patient—therefore, nothing can be done for this patient" is fallacious. The best copers and most effective interveners are themselves optimists who believe that the future can be better, regardless of the prognosis. Such people tend to confront problems directly, redefining salient issues constructively, seeking competent assistance when needed, and selectively addressing themselves to problems that are most alarming and disconcerting.

To help vulnerable patients cope better, one must understand their previous strategies for coping with crises. There is no better way than simply to *ask* how a patient usually deals with problems and concerns. Answers are often very revealing:

"I always ask my sister's advice."
"I tend to pray more than most people."
"I just push everything out of my mind."
"There's no use getting upset. I accept it."
"Sometimes I raise hell with everyone."
"I might drink too much."
"I take the phone off the hook, then hate people for not calling."

Coping strategies will be described more fully in Chapter 3. But coping is a process that combines several different kinds of behavior, with varying mixtures of active and passive strategies, depending on the intended purpose. No strategy works for all problems, but some tend to work better than others, more often. There is also a difference between a *show* of distress, which is a sign of vulnerability, and a type of *behavior* that copes with distress.

Safe conduct for patients is for all seasons and states of being, thick and thin, from initial impact on. Coping with cancer cannot mean greeting each adversity with a smile or a shrug. Everlasting equanimity is something that few healthy people achieve, and should not be expected of cancer patients who undergo successive recurrences or progressive debilitation. Any positive contribution is a boon, not to be disparaged. While complete resolution of all problems is a dream founded on an illusion, distress can be brought to a tolerable level, along with management of principal problems.

Antidepressants, tranquilizers, narcotics, or combinations of drugs are often necessary, and should not be withheld; neither should they replace compassionate care and safe conduct. Almost everyone needs palliation or relief of some sort, regardless of illness, just as an element of being alive and vulnerable. If a patient seeks miracles, it must be done elsewhere, but prudent encouragement to cope in accordance with earlier, lifelong values is a prized act of responsibility.[10] The philosophy that advocates trying anything, "What is there to lose?" is pernicious. Even preterminal patients have much to lose by chasing rainbows. They lose a chance to achieve a compatible, and even an appropriate, conclusion. Relatives can do more by sharing final hours with a dying patient than by desperately reaching for a solution that is not there. Safe conduct never ends.

REFERENCES

1 Weisman, A., *On Dying and Denying: A Psychiatric Study of Terminality*, Behavioral Publications, New York, 1972.

2 Weisman, A., and J. W. Worden, "Psychosocial Components of Lagtime in Cancer Diagnosis," *Journal of Psychosomatic Research,* **19**: 69–79, 1975.

3 Hackett, T. P., N. H. Cassem, and J. W. Raker, "Patient Delay in Cancer," *New England Journal of Medicine,* **289**:1 14–20, July 5, 1973.

4 Robbins, G., M. MacDonald, and G. Pack, "Delay in Diagnosis and Treatment of Physicians with Cancer," *Cancer,* **6**:624, 1953.

5 Rakel, R., and H. Conn (eds.), *Family Practice,* 2d ed., W. B. Saunders Company, Philadelphia, 1978.

6 Oken, D., "What to Tell Cancer Patients: A Study of Medical Attitudes," *Journal of the American Medical Association,* **175**:1120–1128, April 1961.

7 Mount, B., A. Jones, and A. Patterson, "Death and Dying: Attitudes in a Teaching Hospital," *Urology* **4**(6):741–747, December 1974.

8 Weisman, A., "The Patient with a Fatal Illness—To Tell or Not to Tell," *Journal of the American Medical Association,* **201**:646–648, 1967.

9 Weisman, A., "Early Diagnosis of Vulnerability in Cancer," *American Journal of Medical Science,* **271**(2):187–196, 1976.

10 Weisman, A. , "Death and Responsibility: A Psychiatrist's View," *Psychiatric Opinion,* **3**:22–26, 1966.

Chapter 3

The Coping Process

WHAT IS COPING?

Coping may be defined as what one does about a problem in order to bring about relief, reward, quiescence, and equilibrium. This definition contains three essential facets of coping. First, there is a recognized problem from which one seeks relief, respite, and resolution. Second, what one does, or does not do about that problem, constitutes how one copes. Third, there is an outcome, which, however, offers no permanent guarantees about the long-term effectiveness of the coping strategy.

As many other investigators have emphasized, coping is a process, not an isolated set of independent actions.[1] It combines perception, performance, appraisal, and correction, followed by further activity, and directed, motivated behavior. While what one eventually and precisely does may be highly individualistic, general types of behavior, which cover more specific tactics, are called strategies or Copes (see Table 1). Coping does not merely consist of gradually feeling better, or less distressed; it is also important to *know* that what one does or did contributed to that relief or resolution.

It is a mistake to separate cancer-related problems from concomitant

Table 1   General Coping Strategies—Cope

---

1 Seek more information (rational inquiry).
2 Share concern and talk with others (mutuality).
3 Laugh it off; make light of situation (affect reversal).
4 Try to forget; put it out of your mind (suppression).
5 Do other things for distraction (displacement/redirection).
6 Take firm action based on present understanding (confront).
7 Accept but find something favorable (redefine/revise).
8 Submit to the inevitable; fatalism (passive acceptance).
9 Do something, anything, however reckless or impractical (impulsivity).
10 Consider or negotiate feasible alternatives (if x, then y).
11 Reduce tension with excessive drink, drugs, danger (life threats).
12 Withdraw into isolation; get away (disengagement).
13 Blame someone or something (externalize/project).
14 Seek direction; do what you're told (cooperative compliance).
15 Blame yourself; sacrifice or atone (moral masochism).

---

problems too sharply. Cancer does not abolish preexisting problems, but may aggravate far milder concerns. New problems may leap into prominence, with a special urgency, regardless of roots in the past. The "medical plight" is not, therefore, intended to exclude any problem, *provided* that its relevance to cancer and the life of a cancer patient can be identified.

Coping is an everyday occurrence, which scarcely merits attention, unless a problem persists and provokes a measure of abiding distress. For example, if you were asked how you coped with breakfast today, the question would presume a persistent problem about breakfast. Perhaps you must eat quickly in order to catch a train, with the unpleasant dilemma of waiting for food, going hungry, or being late for work. Perhaps the family habitually argues at breakfast, or the food itself is poorly cooked—whatever can go wrong and demand that something be done about it. Without a prior problem, questions about coping are absurd. However, once coping is admitted to be a serious question, then the nature of the preexisting problem can be revised, redefined, or reinterpreted, thereby bringing about different responses designed to permit more effective targeted coping.

Distress is a common, but transient condition. Nevertheless, one looks for problems wherever distress occurs. For example, try to recall an occasion during the past month when you felt any of the following:

Sorrow	Shame
Discouragement	Anger
Resentment	Helplessness
Depression	Embarrassment
Tension	Humiliation
Guilt	Annoyance
Fear	Bewilderment
Indecision	

These feelings, largely unwelcome, will usually distress, dismay, or render a person at least temporarily vulnerable, and may indicate past and present problems. If you felt none of these feelings, even to a slight degree, you are probably very lucky or singularly unresponsive. I am sure that most of these feelings of distress went away spontaneously. Other needed to be coped with, using one strategy or another, usually in 'combination. Resourceful people are always at an advantage, because they are not restricted in the range of strategies to call upon. More rigid people are confined to a narrow body of willful acts and attitudes that reduces diversity to a fixed profile of problematic situations.

Coping with cancer, the specific theme of this book, pertains to the *medical plight:* (1) treatment of the tumor, which is a medical problem, and (2) management of concomitant concerns. The right balance of active and passive coping strategies cannot be prescribed in advance.(The process of coping combines and mixes different types of tactics, depending on the problem and available resources.) ⭐

Many patients freely talk about imminent and actual psychosocial concerns, but just as many defiantly declare that nothing bothers them, except the illness itself, if that. Nevertheless, to know more about coping, we need to know more about their plight. These are sample questions:

1   What problems, if any, do you see this illness creating?
2   How do you plan to deal with them?
3   When faced with a problem you must do something about, what happens? What do you do?
4   How does it usually work out?
5   To whom do you turn when you need help?
6   What has happened in the past when you've asked for help?
7   What kinds of problems usually tend to get you down or upset?

Such queries encourage patients to talk, and help to evaluate how the plight is seen at the moment. But perceptions change; monitoring changes in how one evaluates and corrects a situation is part of the coping process. The sample that a clinician obtains one day may not be predominant the next day. Moreover, few patients are articulate enough to be clear about what they do or do not do, when faced with problems. The semantics of asking about problems, concerns, worries, and so forth would require a separate section.[2]

ILLUSTRATIONS OF COPING STRATEGIES

The act of appraising and generalizing about coping tactics depends on understanding that strategies intermingle, and are seldom found by themselves, unqualified. Then, after proclivities and problems are at least tentatively identified, outstanding tendencies in the drift of coping can be detected. These are the strategies, which are intermediary products of the coping process, between primary intention and completed act. I offer the following illustrations of such tendencies, thereafter referred to as Cope.

Cope 1   Seek more information (rational inquiry).

> *Case 3*   Linda was not one who accepted a harsh fate or a series of obstacles without a struggle. Orphaned at an early age, she was raised by an aunt and uncle. She worked her way through college, and now, aged 23, was married and holding a good job. Then she developed a large neck node, which a local physician said was 'lymphosarcoma,' and that no cure was available. Instead of despairing, Linda took a leave of absence, gathered her medical records, and consulted a noted specialist in Boston. The diagnosis turned out to be Hodgkin's disease, state 2 A, which is very treatable.

> *Case 4*   Paul was a meticulous, even obsessional physicist, who was not reassured to be told "all the cancer is gone" after a groin dissection and wide excision for malignant melanoma. He demanded statistical evidence. The physician agreed, and showed Paul the relevant data. Paul knew that the longer he survived, the better his chances were. Instead of a complete guarantee, he realized that there was a strong probability of cure.
>
>   Three years later, the tumor recurred. Still very rational, Paul coped with the doubtful prognosis as if it were a problem at work that needed to be solved. Later, when he began to decline, Paul complained only that, according to life expectancy tables, he was being deprived of a long life.

Note that neither Linda nor Paul "rationalized" their illness, but did seek rational information about diagnosis and outlook. They coped according to their previous style. Linda was self-reliant and assertive, accustomed to making her own way in the world. Paul sought facts and scorned conjectures, because evaluating probability was part of his profession. They differed in almost every other respect. For example, Linda was forthright and friendly, while Paul was somewhat austere and emotionless.

Cope 2   Share concern and talk with others (mutuality).

> *Case 5*   Doris had been treated for nervousness and fatigue for about a year before a lump in her left breast was found. Several family members had died of cancer, and now Doris and her husband were sure that she faced inevitable death. Both became very agitated, tearful, and bitter about the local physician who had, evidently, mistakenly treated her for another illness, without performing a thorough examination.
>
>   I attempted to reduce their mutual agitation by using a supportive, but very rational approach, pointing out that if their present doctor recommended an operation, he thought that the situation was far from hopeless. Their fear was understandable, but the present alarm was unjustified. Gradually, they became more amenable; Doris had a mastectomy, without complications. However, she continued to ask many questions of almost everyone. While

ostensibly asking for advice, she was seldom reassured for long, nor did she ever seem to act on the advice. It was apparent that Doris hardly listened when people responded, because talking itself relieved distress.

Case 6 Patrick developed a cancer of the colon when he was the same age as his father, who died of the same disease. He had no reason to believe that his fate would be different. Nevertheless, Patrick was hopeful and optimistic. He shared information about the illness with his wife and grown children. They had never let him down, nor had he ever failed to do the best he could. Family solidarity was everything. When he died two years later, his family support had been unwavering. Their grief was deep, but bereavement was short, modest, and, of course, sincere.

Although both Doris and Patrick "shared concern," there was little else they had in common. Doris used other people as a sounding board for releasing tensions, as if she demanded, "Look—listen to me!" For Patrick, talking with others was testimony to deep trust. He did not loosely talk about himself, but had a strong mutual reciprocity with his family. There are, however, other patients who convey a wordless mutuality with a few people, not always including the doctor. Mutuality and trust deserve respect and encouragement, but silence is also a way of coping that needs no emotional catharsis. It is conceivable, furthermore, that Patrick might have confided only in his family, and having done so, gone the rest of his life without talking any further about cancer. Mutuality, to him, meant silent trust; for Doris, mutuality was tension-relieving verbalization.

Cope 3   Laugh it off; make light of situation (affect reversal).

Case 7 Stefan retained high vigor and strong spirit, despite knowing that he had a rapidly growing lung cancer. He joked with men, and flirted outrageously with women, whom he enjoyed embarrassing with flattery and compliments. Nevertheless, he vacillated between unrealistic optimism and morbid preoccupation with suicide, so that it was difficult to be sure about his predominant tendencies. He reported, for example, that one day he looked longingly at his revolver—before deciding that he'd rather die laughing than kill himself.

His only relative was a very frail, younger brother, Joe, who recently came through heart surgery, and was still convalescing when he tried to cheer up Stefan. In a quavering voice, he reassured his brother, "Why, you're looking great! You'll still live to bury me!" Considering Joe's precarious health, a compliment like this was hardly reassuring. Stefan burst out laughing, because neither he nor his brother was likely to live very long, everything taken into account.

Cancer is certainly no laughing matter. Graveyard humor is in exceedingly bad taste. Visitors and staff are usually so solemn and saturnine that laughter is discouraged, and with it goes the gentle humor that makes life tolerable. Joking is usually ill-advised, but some cancer patients do use a wry humor or grim irony, when talking about themselves. No less a personage than Freud, who suffered with cancer for many years, retained his sardonic humor almost until death.[3]

Cope 4   Try to forget; put it out of your mind (suppression).

Case 8   Helen was an unmarried, middle-aged office worker with cancer of the colon. She spent her life caring for an ailing, widowed mother. Her job was routine. She had no friends, never dated, and worked constantly, refusing vactions. She was shy, quiet, and seemed very naïve in all physical matters, even when she developed intestinal obstruction.

She ignored the colostomy, and had to be prodded into learning how to take care of it. There were no questions about cancer, and her only concern was the welfare of her mother. Several months later, when the mother died, Helen was also found to have liver metastases. Again, she ignored her own illness, grieving quietly for her mother. She fell silent. Asked about the future, she said, "Who can tell?" This was less a question than a statement in which she seemed less than interested.

She returned to the hospital when the disease progressed further. While a little confused, she was not anxious, depressed, or discouraged. But rather surprisingly, she told a social worker about having two dreams. In one, she was on an extended vacation in Hawaii, an event, for her, that was as unlikely as flying to the moon. In the second dream, there was a scene in which a funeral service was being conducted for many people at once. They were buried with their heads above ground, and it was not at all sure whether they were, in fact, dead, because a few were talking to each other. In a way, these dreams typified Helen's meager life, which was not that different from death. Her only allusion to cancer over many months was in a letter to an aged aunt. She wrote, "The doctors are still looking for tumors, but I don't think it is very serious." But it was.

Suppression is hardly stupidity, but it may appear to be *selective inattention* for one reason or another, not always because something is intimidating. Helen's plight had been carefully explained to her, but she seemed wholly disinterested in anything except her mother. Filial altruism seemed to guide everything she did. Literally, she had sacrificed her own life for this duty. Suppression and displacement, however, are often observed in patients who readily, even incessantly, talk about other people with cancer, not themselves. One man, for example, whispered to his wife, "Watch what you say. All the other men in this room have cancer!"

Cope 5   Do other things for distraction (displacement/redirection).

Case 9   Marion was an affluent, worldy woman in her mid-50s when she developed breast cancer. During convalescence, she quickly returned to a busy, busy schedule of volunteering, attending parties, or any other occasion that took her out of the house. Previous engagements even interfered with the radiation treatments. She attempted also to play golf again, when it was clearly premature.

She confided that she had been married and divorced three times, before marrying her present husband, a wealthy man at least 20 years older. Among other things, she mentioned that a favorite brother committed suicide years before, and that several other members of her family had been hospitalized for severe depressions. Therefore, it was likely that much of her activity, discontent, and search for immersion in something outside herself fended off fear of depression, and just possibly, prevented suicide. She was very afraid of dying, and very reluctant to disclose anything further about her life.

One cannot be perpetually preoccupied with symptoms and foreboding. Coping by distraction, including displacement of concern to someone or something else, need not be pathological. Indeed, rapid return to activity, especially when coupled with energy and optimism, may be highly beneficial. Morale can be helped by competent performance, joined with a sense of worth, even if the activities seem contrived. Many men and women with a personal history of cancer later volunteer in hospitals or organizations that service cancer patients. Not only do such activities distract, but transform passive coping into a valuable, active strategy. Moreover, some patients compromise between activity and passivity in a substitute distraction. If a patient is prevented from attending the theater, she or he may still keep informed by reading plays, books, or reviews, often in the company of others.

Cope 6   Take firm action based on present understanding (confront).

Case 10   George was a self-made, successful businessman who was found to have an asymptomatic lung cancer, while in the midst of acquiring still more business interests. His response was typical. He began making contingency plans, in the event of recurrence after surgery. He screened potential successors, rewrote his will, and arranged for his widowed mother's continued support. On the other hand, in case the tumor should not return, he also investigated new markets and opportunities. He approached the uncertainty of cancer with the same prudence, decisiveness, and speculative flair that made him so successful in business. He was firm, frank, realistic, and objective. Except for periodic readmissions, it was "business as usual," but without suppression.

Every competent coping pattern, however interlaced with other strategies, requires confrontation, followed by firm and appropriate action. Without it, patients are reduced to avoidance, passivity, withdrawal, equivocation, or impulsiveness. Of course, not every action is appropriate or opportune. Correction is usually necessary, as events unfold. But correction itself is an appropriate action, because it is a desirable way to shape strategy. Never does the patient who uses Cope 6 ignore the reality of the medical plight.

Cope 7   Accept, but find something favorable (redefine/revise).

> *Case 11*   Emma, a 75-year-old widow, discovered a mass in her breast, sought
> out a competent surgeon, and underwent a mastectomy. She accepted the
> personal and medical situation without any apparent alarm. She said that were
> she a much younger, married woman, she could understand why losing a
> breast might be quite distressing. However, it meant little to her, other than the
> discomfort of the operation itself. She compared mastectomy to hysterectomy
> in a postmenopausal woman. The cancer did not escape her attention, but it
> caused no alarm.

> *Case 12*   Unlike Emma and other older women, Sheila was only 45, and still
> married, when diagnosed as having metastatic breast cancer. Mastectomy was
> unlikely to offer lasting benefit. She accepted the prognosis, but added that
> because she and her husband were married while still in their teens, they had
> had the equivalent of a very long marriage. Their children were now grown, no
> longer dependent, and her husband was still young enough to marry again,
> should he want to. She could conceive of remarrying, were the situation re-
> versed.

The effect of Cope 7 is to put a bad situation into a better, more
benign, and acceptable light. Consequently, some examples of 7 could be
mistaken for denial. For instance, a bedridden father of young children was
forced to be in the hospital over Christmas. Despite this sad situation, he
volunteered that he preferred being away from his children, even though he
was always eager to see them; there would be just too much confusion at
home. Reinterpretation is, actually, an excellent mode for rationalizing illness into smaller complaints. One woman said she was short of breath
because the room was stuffy; her poor appetite came from bad hospital
cooking; weakness was due to inactivity, and so on. Conceivably, revising
each of these signs of illness into manageable fractions created something
favorable about the total impact of illness. Cope 7 works best, however,
when combined with Cope 6.

Cope 8   Submit to the inevitable; fatalism (passive acceptance).

> *Case 13*   Henry, aged 75, lived alone on a small pension. His wife was long
> dead, and his five children had dispersed. With few outside contacts, Henry
> seemed content to remain in his room, especially after recovering from a seri-
> ous heart attack, 3 years earlier. When it was found that he had lung cancer,
> and that surgery was indicated, Henry did not protest, because cancer seemed
> to have little importance.
>   During convalescence, Henry became even more inactive. As a result, he
> gained much weight and his diabetes worsened. He told no one about his
> nausea related to chemotherapy, except a social worker who urged him to
> discuss it with his doctor. "Why mention it?" he said. "The doctors are only
> interested in the tumor, not my cough, or that I can't keep food down." Later

on, he commented, fatalistically, "Well, I never counted on living to be a hundred, anyway. Why ask? I get the message." Still later, now feeling bored, "Why postpone? If they want to treat me, O.K., but not too much, please," His attitude was one of resignation, without exhaustion or apathy. He did not want to notify his children, and when asked, spoke only briefly and laconically about his late wife, as if he hardly remembered. His general attitude resembled the restless resignation of a man forced to wait for a train that was late in arriving. He gave up testing his urine. He also gave up eating, then stopped talking, or answering questions. Finally he gave up everything else, and drifted into death.

Cope 8 is generally signified by an air of pervasive inevitability, with or without apathy and indifference. However, it is important to differentiate between apathy and acquiescence. One can cooperate submissively and acquiesce, without apathy, exhaustion, or indifference. As time goes on, however, acceptance and passivity fuse. A weary traveler like Henry was ready to accept anything but prolonged treatment. He had no ties, nowhere to go, because he was at the end of the line.

Cope 9   Do something, anything, however reckless or impractical (impulsivity).

Case 14   At age 39, Joe was still a bachelor, living at home, and working at a very nonessential job in the family business. But it paid enough to support his leisure in bars and at the race track.

Shortly after an operation for malignant melanoma, Joe decided that it was time to get married. However, all the women he knew were pickups from bars or very casual acquaintances. He did remember a young woman he met several years earlier on a cruise. Evidently, she had shown some interest, because they corresponded briefly. Somehow, Joe concluded that they were ideally suited. He then journeyed to another country to see her, and try to arrange a marriage. He passed himself off as a wealthy American businessman, impressing both the girl and her parents. She soon had reason to regret the marriage. For example, he attempted sodomy on their wedding night, trying to force her into capitulation. They slept apart; the marriage was never consummated, and she soon discovered the hoax about his wealthy family. She left, and later obtained an annulment. Joe could not understand why she deserted him, but soon returned to his familiar habits.

Acting out, which is a good synonym for Cope 9, means that someone regularly or impulsively carries out socially unacceptable, potentially harmful acts without heeding consequences or being able to restrain such actions. It is assumed that acting out is prompted by inner conflict or tension. For the most part, patients who are culpable of acting out, and it is considered undesirable, attempt to reduce emotional tension to a manageable level, although there is no lasting resolution of the inciting problem. One man deserted his wife and children shortly after a cancer diagnosis, only to return home, repentantly, a few weeks later.

Cope 10   Consider or negotiate feasible alternatives (if x, then y).

Case 15   Connie developed Hodgkin's disease when she was 34 years old, married 6 years, and the mother of a small daughter. She wondered what the remainder of life held for her, not only whether she would live, but what she had missed. Her husband was quite sympathetic with her dissatisfaction, but cautious. For example, when she considered joining the Peace Corps or the Indian Service, he advised her to think seriously before taking this extreme step, away from home and family. He urged her to consider what she might gain, or lose, patiently listening to other possibilities that Connie was obviously unsuited for. After a few desultory inquiries, her restlessness subsided, as if by considering alternatives, action became less urgent.

Case 16   Thelma was a research worker with an advanced degree. She managed a home, raised two children, and held a full-time job until the symptoms of an ovarian cancer forced her to resign. Within a few months, even taking care of the household was too much. However, she arranged with a neighbor to do shopping and prepare meals, as well as transporting her children to school and back. In exchange she tutored this woman who was taking a belated college course for a degree. The plan worked out well. Thelma felt she was not as useless as she expected to be, and the neighbor got her degree.

Although coping usually requires abundant correction and refinement of the initial course of action, negotiation of alternatives, or weighing one possibility against another, takes place so inconspicuously that patients simply report what they do, not their prior consideration of possibly doing something else. Only when something a little unusual develops does someone realize that the medical plight has prompted a new course of considered action. Connie rued her unfulfilled life before coming to terms with it. Thelma traded her talents and worked out an accommodation.

Cope 11   Reduce tension with excessive drink, drugs, or danger (life threats).

Case 17   Jeff's prominent family ostracized him many years earlier, after his undisciplined behavior led to expulsion from college. He gambled, drank excessively, ate a lot, occasionally brawled, and was often robbed when he frequented dives where homosexual prostitutes preyed on older men. At age 55, he worked as a security guard, and lived with a series of roommates. Mainly, however, his life consisted of whatever turned up at night, which he admitted was somewhat precarious. Nevertheless, liver disease, diabetes, broken bones, and being robbed were apparently worth the price. When he was found to have lung cancer, he feared pain, not death. At no time did he grieve or complain. The excitement and danger he underwent seemed to mean much more than anything related to his health or safety.

Ordinarily, intoxication, overeating, and taking pills for one reason or another hardly qualify as coping strategies, except that using drink, food, and drugs regularly, excessively, and even on special occasions, does relieve tensions. Obviously, the complications of alcohol, obesity, and drug abuse are enormous. However, for people like Jeff, life-threatening behavior or noxious habits is a life style, despite the danger. His character consisted of coping via alcohol, eating, and risky behavior. Not much else mattered. In general, cancer patients who regularly abuse alcohol continue, and do not become abstinent. Abstainers do not turn to drink. However, successful AA members seem to cope very well with cancer, and seldom relapse, perhaps because the famous Twelve Steps of Alcoholics Anonymous are good coping strategies under any circumstances.[4]

Cope 12   Withdraw into isolation; get away (disengagement).

> *Case 18*   Harriet separated from her husband shortly after the birth of their daughter, now 20 years old. They married only to legitimize the pregnancy, and his departure was expected. Nevertheless, Harriet never sought a divorce, hoping that he would return. She shunned overtures of other men, and led a more or less solitary existence. She worked for years in a small restaurant, supporting her daughter, and refusing to see other members of the family, who invited her to visit. She also neglected a growth on her neck until her boss forced her to seek medical care. It was Hodgkin's disease, and amenable to treatment.
>
> Regardless of the good prognosis, Harriet procrastinated, hoping that the tumor would go away. She canceled clinic appointments on the feeble pretext of having to work, or feeling too weak. In fact, her attitude toward treatment was like her feelings about her absent husband. She hoped that he would come back, just as she hoped to get better without doing something about it. Meanwhile, she withdrew into a life of semiphantasy, refusing to establish other relationships.

Like Jeff, Harriet is an exceptional case. But she shows how withdrawal can be almost life-threatening in its totality. Not every person who withdraws is like Harriet, by any means. Milder forms of disengagement after cancer diagnosis are common, because not everyone seeks to share concern or talk things over. There are several types of social withdrawal:

1   Natural loners who keep their distance and enjoy solitude.
2   Retreaters who seek isolation in order to think things through, settle on the next step, muster strength, get perspective, weigh alternatives without distraction, and so on.
3   Vacationers who respond to stress by seeking scenery changes, instead of dealing with a current problem. Vacations seem to legitimize procrastination, but there is also little doubt that going away might mean a wish that every other problem would also go away.
4   Dreamers who live out a phantasy existence, independently of everyday problems and exigencies that require practical solutions. Schizoid withdrawal is a severe example.

Loners say, "I've always faced problems myself. I see no reason to change now." Retreaters say, "I must think things over. It has all happened so fast. I've never been sick before. Maybe I'll call you later on." Vacationers quickly decide to absent themselves. "I've always wanted to see California [Hawaii, the Caribbean, and so forth]." "I haven't seen my sister in ten years. I think I'll stay with her for a while before I come in for that operation." Harriet was also a dreamer, who could maintain a vain hope that her erstwhile husband would return, while excluding all but the most tangential relationships. She also withdrew from tumor treatment, as best she could.

Cope 13   Blame someone or something (externalize/project).

Case 19   Hank was a life-long victim of hard luck. After his parents died at an early age, he lived in a series of foster homes before starting out on his own. Four brothers and sisters died by the time Hank was 30 years old, from accidents, tuberculosis, and cancer. Now Hank himself had lung cancer.

Hank's work history, to put it mildly, was erratic. Typically, he worked in mills, quarries, farms, and factories. But he would either argue with the boss over some grievance, feeling imposed upon, or simply walk off the job, without notice. At one time, he spent about 2 years in a penitentiary for alleged robbery. Later, he was in a state hospital because of alcoholism. Hank now wanted nothing to do with hospitals, institutions, treatment, and, particularly, anything that suggested mental testing. He agreed to casual conversations, however, and what was learned about him came from his many denunciations of foundry work, which caused the cancer, of unsympathetic employers who exploited him, of prison conditions, and of hospital psychiatrists who gave him drugs that endangered his mentality.

Case 20   Mildred blamed her father's infidelity for her mother's early death and her own divorce. She trusted no one, and believed only in the efficacy of prayer. When a cancer caused bowel obstruction, she blamed sickness on constant aggravation at the office. She was forced to take on extra work, she claimed, because younger women spent most of their day in talking about dates, boyfriends, clothes, and similar frivolities.

Life itself is no model of justice, mercy, or equity. Some patients resent cancer as an unfair burden, heaped upon earlier insults and injuries. "It's just one more thing, Doctor." Hank could well be dubbed "psychopathic," but his troubles were always ascribed to nefarious domination or brutal exploitation by people in authority over him. Mildred, too, overpowered by her plight, pictured herself as a martyr for the cause of virtue. But while virtue must be its own reward, it need not be a punishment. Nevertheless, some people cultivate uprightness, cleanliness, austerity, and so forth, as if to protect themselves against misfortune. Then they feel let down when something goes wrong. Not too different are others who consider themselves constantly beset by hostile forces and duplicity in people they are tempted to trust. Cancer is "ideally" suited to represent every misfortune that is worth resenting.

Cope 14   Seek direction; do what you're told (cooperative compliance).

> *Case 21*   Mary worked in a factory at a routine job for 30 years. She had
> known about a mass in her breast for about 10 months. By the time she
> consulted a physician, the cancer had spread to several bones and, presumably,
> to her liver. Her life expectancy was, of course, thought to be very short.
> Chemotherapy was all that could be offered. Nevertheless, when the staff phy-
> sician told her not to worry, she didn't, nor did she ask questions or request
> medication.
>
> Weeks went by. Mary had surprisingly few symptoms. When another
> physician once volunteered that the cancer seemed to have stopped growing,
> Mary quietly responded, very politely, "That's nice. Thank you." She wanted
> to go back to work, but was never insistent, worried, anxious, or depressed
> about her prolonged inactivity. Indeed, she lived far beyond original expecta-
> tions. When transferred to a nursing home, she acquiesced without question,
> and was not at all resigned or apathetic. She was a model patient.

Mary coped by using naïve passivity, which fitted in well with her quiet
optimism. Except for her hopeful attitude and lack of fatalism, she could
well have been classified as calling on Cope 8, or inevitability with surrender. The well-known strategy, "Wait and see," usually involves Cope 14,
combined with suppression (Cope 4).

There are probably a substantial number of patients who are as yet
undiagnosed, and live out their lives without seeking any direction about
obvious symptoms of cancer. Sooner or later, however, almost every cancer
patient yields to pressure of symptoms, or the persuasiveness of friends, and
finds his or her way to diagnosis and treatment. Most patients, therefore,
show some degree of Cope 14. Although many will protest, they still com-
ply. A truly cooperative patient is assumed to be one who follows directions, without insisting on more information than the physician is willing to
offer. Cope 14, however, is also determined by cultural considerations.
Many patients, especially the very poor, are grateful for any attention, sub-
mitting to whatever is asked of them, without question or search for information. This is not so in more enlightened areas where patients hire private
doctors and pay premiums for medical care. Cooperative compliance is not
always recommended, because some patients do not find qualified authori-
ties. To work well, Cope 14 needs to be combined with Cope 1 or Cope 10.

Cope 15   Blame yourself; sacrifice or atone (moral masochism).

> *Case 22*   Joseph was 58 when he developed lung cancer. He had surprisingly
> few complaints, calmly accepting the diagnosis, and regretted the inconve-
> nience he imposed on the staff and his family.
>
> He was a successful businessman, father of four grown children, and
> long-suffering husband of a virago. She humiliated Joseph at every opportuni-
> ty, drank excessively, and antagonized her children, who often pleaded with

Joseph to stand up for himself and even to get a divorce. He would quietly agree, but scarcely raised his voice, despite provocation over many years.

He also seemed to regard the cancer somewhat dispassionately. Just as business success gave him no pleasure, lung cancer caused no pain and no special concern. He was a faithful churchgoer, but felt neither let down by God nor punished for fancied misdeeds. He did not overtly declare that cancer was a punishment, that he felt guilty and now had to make amends. Rather he accepted his illness much as he accepted his punitive wife. As the cancer progressed, Joseph also outraged his children by making his wife the executrix of his estate, although she had shown no evidence of relenting or changing her ways during his illness. Joseph's only explanation was an apologetic remark that he didn't want to hurt her feelings!

Moral masochism is a somewhat arcane psychoanalytic concept that refers to people who victimize themselves, tolerate exploitation without complaint, or volunteer for the dirtiest jobs imaginable.[5] Conversely, the term applies when such people are made uneasy by success or feel guilty when they show any indignation. Joseph certainly would qualify as an outstanding moral masochist, if these criteria are correct. There are also people who implicitly believe in magic, atone for presumed misdeeds, interpret illness and failure as retribution, and sacrifice something valuable or sought-after in an entreaty designed to rectify or reinstate themselves.

Guilt and shame, to say nothing about superstition, obsessional thoughts, and belief in magic, are almost as prevalent in society at large as sadness, anxiety, anger, and fear. Because cancer is commonly regarded as about the worst misfortune that can befall anyone, it is very surprising that so few patients interpret their illness as retribution. Of course, an occasional cancer patient proposes to live a better life, if spared, but this is a form of bargaining, not atonement. Some new patients declare that they smoked, drank, or fornicated too much, not necessarily in that order, but enough to convey the idea that dissipation or disregard of health has led to cancer. Smoking is certainly a better documented cause of cancer than is promiscuity, gluttony, or other forms of misbehavior. However, "I had it coming to me" is heard much less frequently than "I have been working too hard." Patients talk about their theories of causation, without indicating any guilt or contrition. Perhaps cancer itself relieves a bad conscience or attenuates a disposition towards self-blame or shame. If so, then according to this hypothesis, cancer is a somatic punishment befitting a moral crime. The disease would then enable such a person to solve preexisting problems.

COPING AND DEFENSES

The relationship between coping with a problem and defending against psychological conflict has not been satisfactorily worked out. "Defense mechanisms" are almost part of everyday speech, but coping strategies are very new. "A person will cope if he can, defend if he must, and fragment if he is forced, but whichever mode he uses, it is . . . in the service of organization." Haan, whom I quote, considers coping to be an *open system* which permits new information to be assimilated in the service of better accommodation to reality.[6] She regards defensiveness or fragmenting, i.e., regression, as a *closed system* that prevents modification of behavior in response to reality. In other words, according to Haan, coping uses information to regulate and modify behavior in response to a new problem, while calling upon older patterns of defense when first confronting the problem. I do not agree. Entrenched habit or custom are dispositions which may not be the best way to deal with an obstacle. Change in coping, based on what has or has not worked well in the past, leads to a more desirable strategy, while defending implies a kind of rigid repetitiveness, regardless of the problem.

That the interface between external and internal problems is hazy needs no argument, but there are distinct differences between coping and defending, even though both processes may come into action at the same time. A prerequisite for coping is to have a recognized problem which needs to be dealt with. In contrast, most people when they are being defensive do not realize what they are fending off.

How do these differences apply to cancer patients? There is nothing that prevents a patient from coping with a problem, while simultaneously defending against a variety of unspecified problems. Also, what a problem consists of depends on who is defining it. One woman, stuck in a routine job, insisted upon going back to work as soon as possible after her operation. Her doctors considered this unwise and premature, but she was adamant. Another woman, with an equally uninspiring job, decided, following an operation, to take a long-deferred trip to Rome and visit the Vatican. Because she needed chemotherapy, this, too, was thought to be premature. Were these women coping or defending?

The first patient apparently wanted to resume work and stay put; the second patient thought it was time to break her routine. Unsympathetic observers might say that the first woman was compulsively determined to ignore illness and return to business as usual, and that the second woman was impulsively acting out a phantasy, disregarding her treatment. More sympathetic observers would say that the first woman was very conscientious about work and loyal to the job, and that the second woman was very devout and wanted to fulfill a dream important to her faith. Unsympathetic observers would not hesitate to call both behaviors "defensive." Sympathetic observers could call their actions "coping." Defensiveness, or using defenses, means fending off an unspecified problem, and is ordinarily not considered very admirable.[7] Coping is thought to be a good thing to do, provided that the strategy is socially sanctioned, i.e., not reckless, imprudent, revolutionary, or so on.

We could go on, disputing whether these two women are to be praised for coping or blamed for defensiveness, and come to no conclusion—unless we understand the predominant problem that each hoped to deal with by different methods. It turned out that both women had difficult, complaining mothers whom they supported, but detested. "Getting away from mother" was the problem, and their coping strategies, quickly going back to work or visiting Rome, were essentially the same (Cope 5).

In everyday life, we know surprisingly little even about people we know and care most about. We assume a great deal more about their motives and attitudes than may be true. To understand more about coping and defending in patients whom we probably know less about, it is essential to elicit a *primary problematic situation*, about which a patient is trying to do something. To presume that everyone must be concerned about this or that, or that any behavior we disapprove of is defensiveness, is dogmatism.

To understand coping, it is necessary to raise our level of tolerance and to consider what people do, and why, plausibly, they might do it that way, and not another way. Conclusions are always open to correction. When defensiveness is fully understood, as it practically never is, the instigating problem is also understood. Then the behavior is called coping. This is what coping is all about: strategic correction. The 15 coping strategies I have illustrated must be regarded only as a guide, because coping is never permanent. We do not find solutions for human concerns, only temporary truces.

❋ THE BEST AND WORST COPING STRATEGIES ❋

There is no secret formula for good coping that fits everyone with cancer. No two medical plights are the same. Coping is a skill which calls upon other skills suited to the occasion. If one action better prepares a person for the next problem, then whatever works best, works. The key issues are contained in the consequences of any behavior, and how well those consequences fit with a person's prior intentions.[8]

Resourceful people are less rigid in approaching any problem, even though our character consists of well-worn strategies and selective values, distilled from successful, satisfactory, and rewarding resolutions.

But familiarity with a strategy, whether simple or sophisticated, does not always breed contentment or quiescence. If coping is a skill, then it can be cultivated, using the characteristics that good copers exemplify. Good copers with cancer, despite their diversity, seem to follow an implicit set of precepts, which can be translated into positive directives:

1 Avoid avoidance; do not deny.
2 Confront realities, and take appropriate action.
3 Focus on solutions, or redefine a problem into solvable form.
4 Always consider alternatives.
5 Maintain open, mutual communication with significant others.
6 Seek and use constructive help, including decent medical care.

7 Accept support when offered; be assertive, when necessary.

8 Keep up morale through self-reliance or resources that are available.

9 Self-concept is as important as symptom relief.

10 Hope is self-pride, not self-deception.

Good copers understand the difference between being hopeless and powerless. Poor copers usually feel powerless, sick or well. They come into illness having failed in many other ways. Frequently, poor copers are marginal people, with impoverished morale, who feel defeated at the outset. They may insist upon avoidances. "I can do this by myself" may be mere bravado, because it sometimes takes considerable courage to recognize a problem and accept help. Also, poor copers usually deny a great deal, but still have many difficult problems to contend with. They call on wishful thinking, or adopt a very passive attitude, waiting for something to be done. Despite earlier disappointments and pessimism of high degree, poor copers are rigidly compliant, without self-assertion.

The dividing crux between good copers and bad copers is the difference between resourcefulness and rigidity. A second crucial difference is between optimism of a constructive type, and pessimism, which expects replication of earlier defeats. For good copers, cancer is a burden, but not crushing. They confront, do what they can, and call upon available supports, including their own inner resources. They demand and yield selectively, anticipating blunt realities, but knowing that not every problem can be solved. Nevertheless, more problems are solved by awareness and acceptance than by disavowal, avoidance, and denial.

REFERENCES

1 Lazarus, R., *Psychological Stress and the Coping Process,* McGraw-Hill Book Company, New York, 1966.

2 Moos, R., "Psychological Techniques in the Assessment of Adaptive Behavior," in G. Coelho, D. Hamburg, and J. Adams (eds.), *Coping and Adaptation,* Basic Books, Inc., New York, 1974, pp. 334–399.

3 Schur, M., *Freud: Living and Dying,* International Universities Press, New York, 1972.

4 *Alcoholics Anonymous: The Story of How Many Thousands of Men and Woman Have Recovered from Alcoholism,* Works Publishing Inc., New York, 1946.

5 Reik, Theodor, *Masochism in Modern Man,* translated by M. Beigel and G. Kurth, Farrar, Straus and Co., New York, 1941.

6 Haan, N., *Coping and Defending: Processes of Self-Environment Organization,* Academic Press, Inc., New York, 1977.

7 Kroeber, T. C., "The Coping Functions of the Ego Mechanisms," in *The Study of Lives,* R. White (ed.), Atherton Press, New York, 1963, pp. 178–198.

8 Ratner, J. (ed.), *Intelligence in the Modern World: John Dewey's Philosophy,* chap. XV, "Perception, Language, and Mind," pp. 795–836; also, chap. XVI, "Thinking and Meaning," pp. 837–884.

Chapter 4

Coping and Denial

Withdrawal from pain is so natural and spontaneous that its mental analogue, denial, is also expected to be natural and automatic. Thus, if cancer
and its implications are the enemy, then our first reaction is to seek a truce
or use any available means to neutralize the supposed threat, even minimizing danger to the vanishing point. But chronic avoidance is impossible. It is
also somewhat demeaning, because of self-deception.

DENIAL AS A PHASE OF COPING

Denial is how one simplifies the complexity of life. When faced with a
threat from which escape is difficult, denial at least temporarily mutes distress. While downright denial can be harmful, denying itself is a phase of
the coping process. It revises or reinterprets a portion of a painful reality,
avoiding what it threatens to be, and holding fast to the image of what has
been. Therefore, denying has three aims: (1) preserving status quo, (2) sim-
plifying a relationship, and (3) eliminating differences between what was
and will be.

Accepting, affirming, and denying can and do coexist. Anything that reminds us of the bleak, ragged edges of existence needs a fence around it. But coping requires more than a fence.

WHAT IS DENIAL?

Denying has five phases: (1) *acceptance* of a common, public reality between one person and another, (2) *elimination* of an objectionable part of that common field, (3) *replacement* with something more congenial and less threatening, (4) *reorientation* with respect to that revised reality, and (5) *judgment* by an observer that denial is an accomplished fact.[1] Denying is an act within the process of coping. It selectively negates or nullifies a threat, substituting another version of reality. But the fact of denial also requires the judgment of someone else about the person who does the denying.

Denying, like other aspects of coping, is not a once once-and-for-all act that conceals an objectionable reality by a flagrant statement, "It did not or must not happen!" Actually, awareness and denying often run together, crossing over as one emotion or perception gains ascendance and blurs another. For example, crossing over is very prominent during early bereavement. When so much of a survivor's reality has depended for a long time upon another person, it is exceedingly difficult suddenly to accept the fact that death has really occurred. Some survivors catch themselves in the act of denying, but as a rule, only an observer can detect more subtle aspects of self-deception.

Denial is not a "mechanism" that one uses in the sense of using eyes or ears. It is a process that repudiates what cannot be avoided, often by substituting a more familiar, agreeable idea. A 61-year-old garage owner with a newly diagnosed, but very malignant lung cancer, explained that the tumor was like a plug in an automobile gas line. It caused him to breathe hard, cough, sputter, and lose momentum. A blast of radiation would blow out the plug, and clear up the whole problem.

Because repudiation and replacement take place within a social field, often for the sake of someone else, denial is also a transaction. It may be encouraged with the collusion of others. Sometimes a patient denies to a spouse in order to preserve their relationship or to maintain self-esteem. The same patient may, however, talk freely to a nurse or social worker, with whom there is an entirely different social transaction. One woman seemed oblivious to the fact of cancer for about 6 years, according to her daughter, despite several operations and courses of chemotherapy. In response, the daughter dissimulated in order to spare her mother. When the patient died, her daughter said, with much relief, that at least her mother never knew and always expected to get well. She was astonished to learn that her mother had spoken with me many times about the illness, treatment, and downward course, even predicting the approximate date of her death!

Had I not known the mother, and relied wholly upon her daughter, the case would have been a good example of tenacious denial. It demonstrates, however, that denial cannot be diagnosed in the abstract, apart from people in the social field for whom a grim, sad fact might be deeply disturbing. Voluntary withholding is not denial.

Case 23   Pete was 17 when his mother died of pancreatic cancer. But for the two years before her death, Pete and his younger brother only knew that she was very ill, up at night, dozing during the day, and much less active. They had no idea that she might die. Meanwhile, they attended school, dated, played sports, and thrived. About a week before her death, their father took them aside and quietly explained the situation.

Thirty years after, with the perverse irony that nature often uses, Pete himself developed abdominal pain and jaundice, which was first thought to be chronic gall bladder disease. Operation disclosed cancer of the pancreas. He now faced the same dilemma with his two sons, aged 15 and 17. Without any hesitation, Pete decided to keep the fiction of gall bladder disease, and not to tell his sons until near the end. Why ruin a year or two of his sons' lives? They would only grieve, feel helpless, and there was plenty of time for that. In retrospect, Pete appreciated the wisdom of his parents. Had he known, a year of adolescence would have been wasted in powerless grief. Although Pete and his wife knew everything possible about the cancer, they told others only about "gall bladder trouble that would take a long time to cure."

I hesitate to call this conscious act of compassion, "denial." Reality has been avoided, but not revised or suppressed. For the mother and daughter who spared each other for 6 years, and for Pete who followed a pattern set by his parents, coping consisted of dissimulation and redefinition (Cope 7) for the sake of others, but confrontation (Cope 6) for themselves.

Spouses are either well-informed or ill-informed, seldom partially informed. The choice about telling children is highly individual. Some well-informed adults still report that they had no idea about their parent's impending death, despite long, conspicuous illness and progressive deterioration. Many people regret not knowing; others, like Pete, are glad. The proper balance between denial and awareness that equals acceptance cannot be packaged into the proper dosage for everyone. Nevertheless, there is a hypothesis which proposes that anticipatory mourning helps prevent future illness and more severe, but delayed grief in survivors. To the best of my knowledge, neither Pete nor his brother had prolonged or aberrant bereavement.

Case 24   Tim was a hard-working carpenter who kept his wife's room locked after her death 7 years earlier. Neither he nor his children ever spoke about her again. When Tim developed lung cancer, he put himself on a weight reduction diet to account for a 15-pound weight loss, and ascribed his cough to a "bad case of bronchitis." He doubted the diagnosis, but failed to ask for further information, indicating that he needed to know nothing more. When his family complained about being uninformed, Tim simply said that he was just taking treatments, and that his doctors were too busy to talk very much.

One day, a clinic doctor sat down with Tim and his oldest son, who happened to be with him, and explained what was wrong and why Tim had not improved. The information was received in silence, and never mentioned again. Several months later, Tim said that the doctor had told him nothing he hadn't already known. Then he changed the subject and talked about going back to work. When a social worker questioned the feasibility, Tim seemed uncomprehending, saying that he was far too young to consider retiring. His physical condition was precarious enough to require a gastrostomy several weeks later.

Denial is such a complex transaction, involving inferences and observations about a social field, that ratings of denial from slight to major are not apt to measure anything more than predominant tendencies at that moment. Nevertheless, physicians and families often justify efforts to fortify denial, on grounds that a patient might lose hope. It is more likely that their own hope is involved at least to the same degree, and this is not improved by deception.

Cancer patients with higher perceived denial and fewer professed needs to know more are *not* more hopeful. Indeed, they tend to feel more helpless and much less vigorous than people who openly acknowledge their plight. Ironically, the very process intended to foster well-being undermines vitality and collaboration. Patients who state that they need nothing may lull supportive people into tacit withdrawal. Significant others can and do encourage denial, directly or indirectly, by keeping distance and closing off. For example, Tim's daughter took care of him during the final months when swallowing was impossible and a gastrostomy had to be done. He was often incontinent and needed frequent bathing. She could cope only by imagining that Tim was a stranger, not her father, and that she was a professional visiting nurse. It was denial by fantasy, if not self-hypnosis. She knew, of course, that Tim was her father at all times, except that denial and awareness crossed over whenever she had to bathe him or clean the gastrostomy tube.

That denial is not a satisfactory coping strategy was shown once again after Tim's death. His daughter had disturbing dreams about him and was bitter about the treatment, declaring that no one had ever spoken to her father or any family member about what to expect. She denied forbidding the staff to tell Tim about the tests, or that Tim was reluctant to discuss anything with them. True to denial, she protested, "Why, we were a very close family that had no secrets between us!"

The existential event that denial defines depends on how much revision has taken place. The major results of existential denial are anonymity, injury, and death. Sometimes, patients present themselves as "better than good," just to be sure that they are appreciated, not demeaned. If denial be carried to extremes, however, this is not only denial *by* a patient, but denial *of* that patient by others. Identity is lost. The organic becomes everything; the person is nothing. He or she has been annihilated.

THE DIVERSITY OF DENIAL

Denial does not announce itself, nor does anyone deny in the absence of another person who shares the social field in which denial occurs. Judgment of denial is a surmise that an offensive reality has been nullified to some degree, and recast into a different form. One must therefore note what is denied, when it happens, to whom the revealing nonrevelation is expressed, and the form in which negation is conveyed. Suppression and avoidance are not denial, but Tim's daughter and her siblings blamed the hospital for not telling Tim what the family had forbidden them to do. In terms of defensiveness, this behavior is projection; as a coping strategy, it is Cope 13.

Defenses are processes that exploit denial, negating facts as well as feelings. Like Proteus, denial assumes many guises and goes by various names:

Rationalization
"I'm really in great shape physically. Sure, I've lost about 25 pounds, but I was too heavy anyway. And what's more, I haven't been hungry, either!"

"I'm sure that if something serious was wrong, my doctor would have told me, and he hasn't. I'm willing to leave things like that up to him."

Displacement
"No, I can't tell you what the trouble was when I first came in. As I recall it, I had been working very hard, but was I sick? Not at all, if you mean was I sick to my stomach, nauseated, or something like that. I guess that the treatments take so long and are so strong that naturally, I'm pretty tired out."

Euphemism
"You see, I had this little growth around my bowels, no bigger than the end of my thumb, maybe smaller. But the doctor took it off, and hooked up the ends of my intestine. And that's about all there is to say."

"I've always had a tendency to get warts. This one turned out to have a deeper core. Now look, all this skin has been removed just for a wart!"

Minimization
"The doctor told me that this sore on my lip was just beginning to turn malignant. That means it might have become cancerous in time, but it didn't."

Self-blame
"No, nothing is wrong with my lung, at least that I remember. But I've got to give up smoking, he says, and I guess that means drinking, keeping late hours,

running around. It's just no good, living it up like I do. Maybe I can give up gambling, too. If I can settle down to a more regular life, I'll be okay."

Compartmentalization
"I can't see what my hip trouble has to do with cancer treatment. That tumor was taken care of a long time ago. These drugs make me sick all over. I don't think I need them. Now they tell me I have a fractured hip. That's like an accident that happened to my aunt who fell down, crossing the street. It has nothing to do with that tumor."

Obviously, before the diagnosis of denial is made, it is necessary to know what a patient has been told, how it was phrased, what was understood, and whether the information was retained, without distortion. These few examples show how little information is accurately absorbed, without being processed through wishes, inferences, and suppositions. The names I have given are less important than recognizing that denying can deflect practically anyone from clear perception and interpretation of the medical plight.

Not only is there endless diversity in denial but there are different degrees or, as I prefer, *orders of denial*.[2] It is easy to recognize three such orders, at least as far as cancer patients are concerned:

1   *Repudiation* of the true diagnosis or fact of illness
2   *Dissociation* of the diagnosis, which is conceded, from its implications or secondary manifestations
3   *Renunciation* of decline, deterioration, and impending demise, despite full knowledge of diagnosis and its relation to subsequent events

Examples of these orders of denial are:

Repudiation (First-order denial): A man whispers to his wife, "Everyone in this room has cancer except me!" Another man says, "I have a stubborn infection, and I won't believe anything else."

Dissociation (Second-order denial): A man with lung cancer complains, "I know that my lung is cancerous, but why do I cough so much?"

Renunciation (Third-order denial): A woman who had received all the chemotherapy and radiation she could tolerate expresses relief, "Now that treatment is over, I'll just wait and see. I guess I'll be sick for a while yet, but maybe I ought to think about retiring from my job anyway."

MIDDLE KNOWLEDGE

At no time during the course of cancer is the mixture between awareness, acceptance, and denial seen more vividly than in the phenomenon of middle knowledge. It happens this way. A patient with advanced cancer suddenly behaves and talks as if nothing is wrong, despite full knowledge of the illness and its manifestations. Some patients begin to talk about going back to work, starting a new business, or, if one knows the background, returning to a point in earlier life when a critical decision was made. Now, however, such patients imply that, given a second chance, another decision might be made which would significantly alter later life, of which, in reality, very little remains. One woman, for example, gave up an important executive job in a small city in order to permit her husband to take a better position in Boston. Although she had misgivings about the move years before, she still considered it a wise decision (Cope 10). Nevertheless, during the waning days of her life, she brought up the question of going home again, starting a new business, and leaving her husband.

Because middle knowledge, which means knowing and not knowing at the same time, comes when a patient is very ill, and without many resources, declarations about "beginning again" have a poignant irony. More specifically, middle knowledge seems to be most evident in response to equivocation in what doctors say or propose doing. Consequently, out of confusion and reveries, I suppose, a patient opts for what might have been, and in view of the prevailing atmosphere of indecision, visualizes another opportunity.

Middle knowledge is not found only in very sick patients. It may occur in potential or actual survivors who cannot believe that death is near. A mother whose 10-year-old son was being kept alive by mechanical means had been told that cerebral death already occurred, despite artificial heart and lung movements. Nevertheless, each day during her vigil, she would still talk to the child about his playmates, as if he heard and understood. Since determination of death amid artificial support systems is a prime instance of professional equivocation, the unfortunate mother might be forgiven for what, under other circumstances, could be called "delusional" behavior.

Then there are patients who shift back and forth so quickly between awareness, acceptance, and denial that the observer is never quite sure what is understood.

> I'm feeling fine these days. The treatment really seems to be working. I plan to rest up awhile, maybe a week or two, then it's back to the office. In fact, the only thing bothering me just a little is this dragged-out feeling. And I still can't eat very well. Maybe it's just the medicine. Maybe it hasn't had time enough to work. The doctor tells me to eat a little bit at a time, so I won't vomit, without trying a full meal. But I can't even do that. I get very despondent. At night, I don't or can't sleep. I really don't think there's any treatment for me. The doctors just talk. They must know better. But I go on, day after day. It's pretty rough, I tell you!

With almost one breath, this patient goes from high optimisim to deep discouragement. Where does denial begin and end? Presumably, denial pertains to his initial optimism, but what if the prognosis is actually better than the patient reports at the end? Denial does blunt harsh reality, but how does one describe a pessimistic distortion? The person who always manages to snatch defeat from the jaws of victory by finding a negativistic flaw is not unfamiliar. It is a defense against tempting the gods by feeling too good. It is also a denial of facts. If we are willing to believe that denial works in *both* directions, nullifying bleak and pleasant facts alike, then we can explain why some patients who are disposed to deny optimistically do very well, while others who deny will feel deep distress and lapse into helpless dismay.

There is no reason to expect a smooth transition from early denial toward pure acceptance (see Figure 1). Human nature does not work that way. Denial is, of course, more common among patients who are newly diagnosed, and less common among those who have been under treatment for a longer period. Patients who deny initially tend to reach a balance between acceptance and repudiation of illness and its consequences. Denial usually yields to reality testing. But occasional doubts and misgivings can disrupt the equilibrium between denial and acceptance at any time. Others seem to show back-and-forth movement across an imaginary boundary between Yes and No, vacillating and compromising their perceptions and coping. In general, however, those patients who show conspicuous vacillation and indecision also deny more emphatically, and cope less effectively. Reality testing means that we not only test reality as it is commonly construed, but that we are tested by reality, as privately defined.

DIAGNOSIS OF DENIAL

If denial is an indispensable phase of coping, how important is its diagnosis? Why not just assume that everyone has an individualized mixture of acceptance and repudiation, titrated to comfort, and let it go at that?

For practical purposes, leaving subtleties aside, the diagnosis of denial is the denial of diagnosis, i.e., first-order denial. Beyond this point, clini-

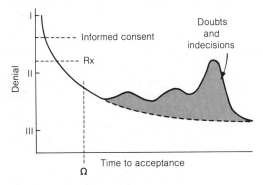

Figure 1   Acceptance of cancer.

cians tend to overlook more elusive variants. My own preference, however, is to pursue denial everywhere. Self-deception not only causes much mischief, but a significant part of psychotherapeutic intervention must include "undenying."[3] An innocent denial may easily be called "selective inattention," but a flagrant denial may have dire, unfortunate consequences. A woman who ignores or denies a growing breast lesion until it fungates, bleeds, and is beyond treatment, and even then continues to deny the need for treatment, is a barely living witness to the effects of avoidance or denial.

Denial of consequences, i.e., second- and third-order denial, can conjure up a half-world of lies and subterfuge that alienates people. If coping equilibrium is heavily weighted with denial, then there are few resources to call upon. The patient is, therefore, dangerously compromised.

PT.: I guess I'm all right now, Doc. Nothing to worry about, is there?

DR.: It sounds as if you've been worrying anyway. What can you tell me about it?

PT.: Well, to tell the truth, I was afraid you might have found something serious.

DR.: Such as?

PT.: Cancer?

DR.: I think you already know that we did find tumor cells after the test, and that's why we need to treat you. That's why we're meeting today— to talk things over.

PT.: Then I do have cancer, after all! I had a notion. . . .

DR.: Yes, that's true. But it may not be as serious as you seem to feel.

PT.: But I have cancer, don't I?

DR.: You also have the idea that having cancer means there is nothing more to do. I want you to understand that this is wrong. This condition can be treated, and with your permission, you will be treated, just as thoroughly as we can.

PT.: Oh, I see. Then even if I have cancer, there's nothing to worry about— just take treatment, and I'm okay?

DR.: I certainly don't want you to worry needlessly. I don't think that ever helps, but this is not a trivial matter any more than it is a hopeless matter. Treatment is necessary, but even afterward, I want you to be checked from time to time, to keep an eye on things. But it's as wrong to say that now everything is okay as to feel like giving up.

In this brief excerpt, the physician provides accurate information, shares concern, nips denial in the bud, and emphasizes positive treatment. Note that the patient tends to twist information into a negation, encouraging the doctor to minimize the condition. However, the physician insists on the diagnosis, follow-up, and a balanced attitude, also permitting the patient to ask questions by answering them accurately and judiciously.

Few cancer patients are without any doubts or qualms and so may resort to denial later on.

PT.:   Why do I have so much trouble walking? That can't be because of my chest condition, can it?

DR.:   What kind of trouble do you have in walking?

PT.:   I stagger a bit, like I'm dizzy or just weak in the legs. All pooped out. I get short of breath. My main trouble is climbing stairs; that's what I'm talking about. Did the x-ray show anything?

DR.:   Yes, it showed that some of the tumor cells have spread in spite of the treatments, but I'll have to check you to find out why you're so pooped out.

PT.:   My God! Just last weekend I felt so good that I started to paint the upstairs hall. Maybe I overdid it, because that was when I noticed how out of condition I was. I haven't had much exercise, you know. Maybe I strained some muscles in my legs, that's all.

DR.:   No, it's probably more than a muscle strain. Painting the hall may have been too much, but it didn't cause what the x-ray shows. The cancer cells are more active than I hoped at this stage. Now we must go on to other treatment, which may work better.

PT.:   In other words, I must rest more?

DR.:   Not at all. Rest when you need to; work when you can. But let's be clear about the facts. Now about that weakness. . . .

DENIAL AND INFORMED CONSENT

Recent emphasis on human studies in the federal and private sectors of medicine has made informed consent a most controversial issue.[4] In principle, practically all physicians are in favor of fully informing patients about treatment and diagnosis, including the risks of treatment. In practice, however, many physicians resent such supervision. Instead of refusing outright, they flood patients with arcane information about real and remote risks, couched in language that only a fellow professional understands. This, of course, is a travesty on genuine informed consent. Nevertheless, patients still sign documents they cannot understand, simply because they are encouraged to be docile and compliant. Having obtained a signature, physicians are then complacent about observing regulations.

Genuine informed consent represents a patient's rights, and furthers the doctor's interests as well. It is all too common to find patients who have, ostensibly, been informed about an operation or procedure, and then subsequently deny that they knew what was about to or might happen. When does the denial begin and end—after the procedure, before, or at the time of so-called informed consent? The question of who is denying what to whom before a procedure can very easily be answered by using the sample questionnaire in Table 2 a day or so *after* the primary pitch by the physician.

Few patients are unequivocally clear about their diagnosis, treatment, and expectations. But lacunae or gaps in information can be filled.[5] Informed consent would then be genuine, and not a perfunctory misnomer

Table 2 Sample Questionnaire

1 What is the name of your condition? _____

2 Do you now have enough information about the condition and the treatment?

___Yes   ___No   ___Wasn't told anything, except_____

3 Would you like to know more?

___Yes   ___No   ___Uncertain

4 What else would you like to know about?

___Whether I have cancer
___Treatment I'll get
___Outcome of treatment
___Risks of different treatments
___How much it will cost me
___When I can go back to a regular routine
___If I can work again ·
___What happens when the treatments are over

5 The doctor explained that the treatments are mainly expected to:

___Cure
___Help a lot
___Help but may have uncomfortable reactions
___Get better knowledge about my illness
___Have no certain effect but it won't hurt or cause new trouble

6 I agree to the new treatment or procedure because I know there is no sure cure for my illness.

___Yes   ___No   ___Uncertain

7 I am also aware that some effects of the new treatment or procedure carry a risk, and that it is possible to be harmed in some respects, without really helping me.

___Yes   ___No   ___Uncertain

for confused consent. If a patient later protests about not knowing what was going to happen, we are probably dealing with someone who did not want to know, expects things to remain as they were, or cannot accept the fact of diagnosis without resorting to unproductive denial. In a corresponding sense, few physicians could persistently inform by not informing, and then deny that their patients have been kept in ignorance.

THE PRICE AND VALUE OF DENIAL

Denial waxes and wanes. Because hard denial is uncommon, the phenomenon would scarcely be worth emphasizing, were it not that cancer patients who confront their concerns with positive strategies do better in all respects. Their needs are less, demands are fewer, genuine support is more available.

In contrast, where denial predominates, distress fails to be contained for very long. Indecision, pessimism, and helplessness grow, despite protestations about needing no one or nothing. Unmitigated denial almost always produces isolation from people whom a patient needs most, even if its purpose is to preserve a relationship. True enough, an unreconstructed, jocular denier kids around with doctors and nurses, seemingly needing nothing but their approval. For patients in whom denial covers fear of being harmed by doctors and nurses, good will and good humor may be reassuring. For the staff, an unassertive, uncomplaining patient frees them to take care of other people. But this idyllic existence is seldom realized. Denial breeds more denial, and then indifference. It is only humane to encourage patients to know more about themselves, because strategies of avoidance wear out faster than confrontation. There is only one exception to this recommendation: Once in a while, a cancer patient postpones treatment for such a long time that real treatment is impossible. Only palliation can be offered. If this patient now approaches terminality, still spinning out a fictional world in which all is well, or soon will be, and if the family conspires to conceal the true situation, nothing is to be gained by insisting upon "facts." The purpose of minimizing denial, after all, is to help patients deal better with consequences. When the only consequences are pain relief, quietude, and shortly death, let it be in comfort and dignity.

REFERENCES

1 Weisman, A., and T. Hackett, "Denial as a Social Act," in *Psychodynamic Studies in Aging: Creativity, Reminiscing, and Dying,* S. Levin and R. Kahana (eds.), International Universities Press, New York, 1967, pp. 79–110.

2 Weisman, A., *On Dying and Denying,* Behavioral Publications, Inc., New York, 1972, pp. 66–74.

3 Weisman, A., "Confrontation, Countertransference, and Context," *International Journal of Psychoanalytic Psychiatry,* 1(4): 7–24, 1972.

4 Kessenick, L., and P. Mankin, "Medical Malpractice: The Right To Be Informed," *University of San Francisco Law Review,* 8: 261–281, 1973.

5 Francis, V., B. Korsch, and M. Morris, "Gaps in Doctor-Patient Communication," *New England Journal of Medicine,* 280(10): 535–540, 1969.

Noncoping and Vulnerability

Nature's ingenuity in finding ever new ways to inflict suffering upon humanity is seemingly unlimited. That human beings are vulnerable and have only limited resources to combat, control, or neutralize distress scarcely needs proof. But some people cope with problems better than others, although no one, of course, is wholly invulnerable. Unfortunately, not every patient manages to cope with the extra burden of an illness reputed to be so difficult to control. At least a third of newly diagnosed cancer patients have substantial distress during the impact period of their illness, when presumably the outlook is brightest. It seems self-evident that when distress is intense, coping is least effective. The more vulnerable one is or feels, the fewer resources are available.

Distress is difficult to measure and evaluate. Like pain, it is vivid, private, and almost impossible to describe adequately. The concept of "vulnerability" is intended to designate different types, degrees, and fluctuations of distress over time. Because it is inversely related to effective coping, vulnerability is also an implicit measurement of noncoping.

VULNERABILITY AND TYPES OF DISTRESS

Vulnerability is the other side of coping well, and has three specific meanings:

    1   An immediate, distressing mood
    2   A tendency or disposition to behave in ways typical of that mood
    3   An effort to translate the inner, private feeling into more explicit verbal and nonverbal "distress signals"

There are, of course, many feelings or moods that come and go, swirling around us, namelessly, leaving no distressing residues. In fact, only emotional extremes have names, such as depression, anxiety, fear, anger, loneliness, and so forth. They last long enough to become nouns. A disposition to behave in certain ways related to a persistent mood is not only the "motion" part of emotion, but seems to represent a style of expressing or coping with the distress generated by an inner mood or attitude.[1] Such behavior is expressed in words or actions that help an outsider understand what is going on or about to happen.[2] It is part of the process of communication about noncoping. For example, a hopeless person talks about futility, which means, in brief, "There is no use trying to do anything." An embittered patient complains about being mistreated or victimized. By listing grievances truculently, one can surmise about an inner state, much as we guess that a person is thirsty when he or she says, "I want a drink of water," and shows a disposition to look for a water fountain.

This concept of vulnerability permits us to identify certain types of distress over time. Like a fever, distress can also be measured, regardless of its type. It does not signify that one is vulnerable to something in particular, but only that distress signals have been read or reported.

The link between laboratory and everyday life is still too tenuous to permit a firm correlation between, say, catecholamines and a specifically distressing emotion and its emergent behavior. Investigators know about a few neurohormones that interact. Also, the psychodynamics of conflict and threat are partially understood. But hormones are probably only the substrate of individual feelings, and psychodynamics refer to actions, not emotions. Psychodynamics are the psychological justification for aberrant behavior, not its explanation.

At present, we know some grammatical rules about conflict, and have a partial alphabet of hormones, but the lexicon of human distress is largely unwritten. Save for poets and novelists, no one fluently speaks the language of emotional distress and vulnerability.

In their study of mood and temperament, Wessman and Ricks[3] found some consistency among different men who regard themselves as "happy" or "unhappy." For example, happy men tend to be self-possessed, optimistic, confident, and successful. They have a purported purpose in life. Whatever that purpose happens to be, fulfillment outweighs disappointment. In effect, they are successful copers, with minimal vulnerability.

In contrast, unhappy people have a poor sense of self-esteem, no continuity of purpose, and frequently are disappointed with their performance. Instead of being sure and confident, they are shaky about self-esteem and self-concept. In short, they cope poorly, and presumably are highly vulnerable.

Obviously, happiness is hardly a good measure of the worth of one's life. Theoretically, happiness should be the ratio between successes and failures, or between enduring satisfactions and frustrations. But the very notion of happiness is something that only unhappy people tend to talk about. Genuinely competent, fulfilled people find the idea a little odd. Moreover, many people manage to cope effectively with major problems, feel confident in various situations, have a fairly good opinion about themselves, and are thought well of, almost all of the time by others whom they respect, need, or love. Still, they would not generally describe themselves as "happy," perhaps because the term suggests a kind of sunny disposition which implies an insensitivity to the woes of the world. I would prefer to call such people, "low vulnerability, high coping effectiveness, strong morale."

Stable, effective people are not always very happy, in the usual sense of complacent optimism. Nor does happiness assure invulnerability to distress, danger, or mortification. Even very unhappy, melancholic people can cope well, and are not bound over to a prison of distress. It is not necessary to be "happy" to cope well. While cancer patients are generally far from happy about their plight, distress can be kept within bounds, so that distress signals are few. As a result, we infer that they cope in a reasonably effective way. Therefore, to assume gratuitously that the fact of having cancer always creates anxiety or depression simply does not fit with how most cancer patients feel. Their burden may be great, but it is not a bag of rocks.

Perhaps it is the wearing effect of the psychiatric vocation, but when a patient insists that he or she is "very happy," I presume that they are anything but happy, or even satisfied with their ability to cope. Usually, they are resigned to disappointments, so that vulnerability is kept in check, or else they have identified their purpose in life with what is expected of them.

Emotional variability, even to extreme peaks and valleys, may be the price paid for sensitivity, empathy, or capacity to see life from many viewpoints. Stodgy people may be better off, but the ultracomposed, cool, collected person may be ill-prepared for the threat imposed by cancer. Their emotional equilibrium may demand physical intactness and psychosocial rigidity. When challenged, it may falter. When threatened, it may fail. Janis found that very unanxious, apparently sturdy, preoperative patients were at

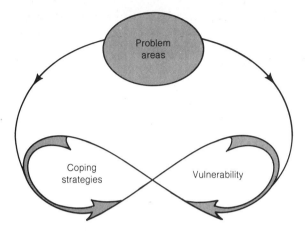

Figure 2 Psychosocial effectiveness.

somewhat greater risk for postoperative problems than their more apprehensive brothers.[4] They tend to feel victimized, or at least misled by physicians, contrary to fact.

It is questionable whether anyone ever gets accustomed to suffering,
and thus is better prepared to deal with it. When predicting emotional
distress in cancer patients, people who are no strangers to misfortune become more distressed than patients from higher social classes who have had
opportunities, resources, support systems, and coped better with problems
in the past. Aged people who, in growing older, have lost families and
friends are not immune to grief and suffering, until or unless they have
developed other, more effective ways of coping.

Psychosocial effectiveness is not a simple equation, but a complex of
forces. Vulnerability, which is a global measure of distress, is only one
aspect of total effectiveness (see Figure 2).

VARIETIES OF VULNERABILITY

Like the endless detail of individual coping strategies, emotional distress is
very personal and idiosyncratic. Feelings are often too deep for words.
Observers, however compassionate, are forced to generalize from a few
signs and signals. Nevertheless, demands of research require measurement
of distress from patient to patient across a span of time. This is a task
somewhat like comparing and measuring the amount of grief in a series of
new widows.

Words convey more than we want at times, but less than we might
wish. To recognize a signal does not mean that we always understand and
can pull discrete observations together. For example, a middle-aged woman
recently learns about having an inoperable cancer. She weeps and smiles at

Figure 3 Omega vulnerability rating scale.

	4	3	2	1
HOPELESSNESS	No hope for recovery	Doubtful regarding recovery	Cautious	Confident regarding recovery
TURMOIL	Highly agitated	Very restless	Fidgety	Calm and composed
FRUSTRATION	Very frustrated; angry over plight	Moderate frustration and anger	Irritable; mild frustration	Feels problems are being adequately handled
DEPRESSION	Very depressed and dejected	Sad; moderately depressed	Mild depression	Not at all depressed
POWERLESSNESS	Feels overpowered; unable to initiate effective action	Not sure if help can help	Needy but able to ask for help	Resourceful and self-sufficient
ANXIETY	Panicky; feels overwhelmed	Frightened, with specific fears	Uneasy; qualms	Feels safe and in little danger
EXHAUSTION	Exhausted; too tired to care	Fatigued and somewhat apathetic	Tired but still cares; seems engaged	Zestful and engaged

	4	3	2	1
WORTHLESSNESS	Worthless; not okay and never will be; undeserving	I'm not okay; feels flawed and inadequate	I'm okay but I goof-up, make mistakes	I'm okay; strong self-regard
ABANDONMENT	Feels abandoned and rejected	Lonely and isolated	Feels somewhat neglected	Feels cared for and well looked after
DENIAL	Avoids speaking word "cancer" or its equivalent	Admits diagnosis and illness, but denies implications	Uncertain or uses euphemism	Correct perception of illness and related problems
TRUCULENCE	Feels victimized, bitter, mistreated by caregivers	Has doubts and serious questions regarding care and treatment	Believes that only "adequate" care is being given	Feels that very good care is received. Very positive attitude to caregivers
REPUDIATION OF SKO	Rejects or antagonizes sources of support	Mild rejection of others; somewhat sullen	Accepts help grudgingly	Gladly accepts sources of help and support
TIME PERSPECTIVE	Closed; no tomorrow	Only a day at a time	Cautious about future; wait and see	Unlimited; foresees future as if no illness

the same time, a curious combination, as if her feelings had been frozen while conversing with friends. Actually, she likes people who can make her laugh, and tries never to be depressed. She does admit to being lonely, now more than ever. Her only relative lives halfway across the country. She is afraid of treatment and of dying alone. Once in a while, she gets angry about being kept waiting for information, and then overreaches herself in being pleasant with nurses.

Ironically enough, the very complexity of vulnerability in this woman is common. I cite her case only to introduce the Index of Vulnerability (see Figure 3). It was devised to express common types of distress and easily recognized distress signals. Of course, it is incomplete, listing only 13 of 52 variables of vulnerability, depending on intermediate degrees, with contrasting attitudes. The signals which can be rated and scored are called "vulnerability variables".

VULNERABILITY VARIABLES

The following descriptions apply only to the most extreme belief or behavior, which rate "4" on the vulnerability scale:

Hopelessness: Patient believes that all is lost, effort is futile, that there is no chance whatsoever.

Turmoil and perturbation: Patient is visibly tense, restless, anguished, and agitated.

Frustration and fractiousness: Patient is irritable, quarrelsome, angry about being sick or unable to find relief.

Despondency and depression: Patient is dejected, tearful, withdrawn, and often inaccessible, speaks in broken phrases and brief responses.

Helplessness: Patient feels powerless to change anything, too weak to struggle, overcome by events, tends to surrender.

Anxiety and fears: Patient has specific fears and dread; may feel doomed or on the verge of panic.

Exhaustion and apathy: Patient feels depleted, defeated, indifferent, and worn out.

Worthlessness: Patient feels at fault, ascribes illness to weakness, flaws, or failure.

Isolation and abandonment: Patient is lonely, feels ignored, uncared for by anyone.

Denial and avoidance: Patient speaks and acts as if ignoring or minimizing threatening aspects of illness.

Truculence: Patient is embittered, feels victimized, mistreated, or put upon by someone or something beyond control.

Repudiation of significant others: Patient rejects or turns away from potential sources of support, usually family or friends.

Closed time perspective: Patient foresees a very limited or nonexistent future.

WHAT CAN GO WRONG BESIDES PHYSICAL DECLINE?

Vulnerability implies noncoping, but there are degrees of noncoping. Moreover, despite patients' protests, many other concerns require coping, besides physical disability. Naturally, like a brief fever, there are cancer patients who heal quickly, leave the hospital, and go about their business with few symptoms and no lasting dismay. Others have persistent signs of cancer treatment, but gradually adapt themselves, with virtually no change in routine. They, too, cope well. Nevertheless, there are some who feel irreparably damaged and destined to deteriorate. Furthermore, vulnerability is not directly proportional to the degree of serious illness. Distress and disease do not keep pace. Noncoping can be found even during remissions. At every stage, patients can be afflicted with nonphysical vulnerability.

The central core of vulnerability is a condition of helpless uncertainty. I call it *existential despair.* When vulnerability variables are factor-analyzed by appropriate statistical procedures, they sort themselves into four clusters or "factors" around a nucleus of depression and powerlessness, which seemingly infiltrates or penetrates almost every type of distress. Depression and powerlessness, of course, need not be extreme, but only pervasive. I do not believe, however, that every cancer patient is simply anxious or depressed; people are too complex to sloganize about them.

The four clusters are called annihilation (hopelessness, anxiety, closed-time perspective), alienation (abandonment, isolation, repudiation, worthlessness), endangerment (frustration, turmoil, truculence), and denial, which is almost an independent factor. Together, these factors comprise the existential plight, which means concern about life and death. Existential despair is not easily detected, because not every patient admits to a degree of depression and powerlessness, especially those who cope well enough to have low vulnerability scores.

As Figure 4 shows, vulnerability factors are not locked in separate compartments, but readily fluctuate and interpenetrate. In extreme form, i.e., when vulnerability is high, patients may, however, feel helpless and uncertain about who they are, who can be relied upon, how to get along. In contrast, when vulnerability is low, self-esteem is correspondingly high, relationships are strong, problems are accepted frankly, and coping is done well. The advantage of factor-analyzing vulnerability is that it offers structure for the medical plight, which can then be dealt with more effectively and directly than merely talking about amorphous, unspecific distress. Cancer patients themselves can also be differentiated according to their most prevalent vulnerability factor.

Annihilation: A cancer patient who feels anxiety, hopelessness, and closed time perspective doubts survival itself. The future is no longer a limitless vista. It must be measured by drops and days. Except for vanishing

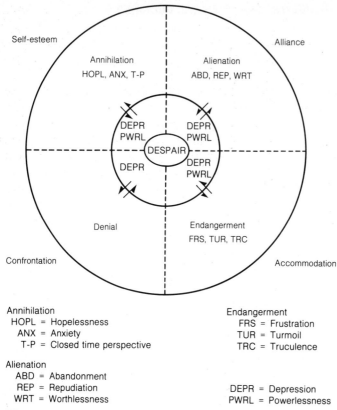

Annihilation
HOPL = Hopelessness
ANX = Anxiety
T-P = Closed time perspective

Endangerment
FRS = Frustration
TUR = Turmoil
TRC = Truculence

Alienation
ABD = Abandonment
REP = Repudiation
WRT = Worthlessness

DEPR = Depression
PWRL = Powerlessness

Figure 4 What can go wrong besides physical decline?

memories and dollops of denial, self-regard is drastically diminished. The disease takes over. Symptoms crowd out every other consideration. The patient feels like a meaningless zero.

Alienation: If annihilation is characterized by apprehension and anxiety, then alienation (abandonment, isolation, repudiation, and worthlessness) is found typically among patients with very conspicuous depression. Those who usually depend much on others are very sensitive to wavering support from family, friends, and professionals. They may expect support but receive little or not enough. They may not expect support and find the prophecy fulfilled. The latter group is also likely to feel worthless, because so much of what we think about ourselves depends on the response we get from others. Frequently, alienated patients repudiate efforts to get closer, lest need be too naked. This usually perpetuates isolation because helpful people, feeling rebuffed, will then tend to draw away.

Feelings of alienation are sometimes fended off by bravado. "I must handle things in my own way. I don't need or want any help." Fear is usually more acceptable to others than alienation, because isolated people withdraw (Cope 12).

Endangerment: Patients who feel in danger may also be irritable, suspicious, embittered, and occasionally very angry, indeed. Endangerment, in fact, means inner resentment about the total plight ("endo-anger"). They refuse to participate, and may even break off treatment because of some real or imagined grievance. "I don't like the effect of this medicine. No one told me about it, and I don't think I need it anyway!" Fortunately, at least for the purpose of investigation, not every patient who feels endangered is angry enough to hang up or walk away. Nevertheless, patients who consent to follow-up interviews frequently feel that even minor inconveniences are major demands. They complain about schedules, parking, waiting, or following treatment protocol. Their attitude is that doctors have somehow cornered or trapped them into an experimental program in which they have no confidence.

Endangered patients, like an endangered species, think of themselves as objects preyed upon. If and when they deteriorate, the illness is misconstrued to be an act of victimization (Cope 13).

> *Case 25* Olga was an aggressive, abrasive woman who successfully ran her husband's business since his death many years before. She smoked at least three packages of cigarettes daily, and was not unduly alarmed to learn that she had lung cancer. However, she resented even the most gently phrased personal questions, and refused psychological testing. She was brusque at her best; unnecessarily rude at her worst. She wondered if the social worker was merely concerned about her ability to pay (she was very affluent), or if the psychiatrist was there to test her sanity.

Denial: A modicum of denial is part of every coping strategy and defense. While it is an emergency response which may not work very well for long, "No, no, it can't be so" is but one form of denial. Most patients are more artful about denial, and as a result, denial permeates other aspects of their life.

> *Case 26* Jacob retired about 2 years before developing lung cancer. He puttered around the house where he and his deaf, withdrawn wife lived since their marriage. Two sons also lived at home, but went their own way, neither asking nor giving very much. Although Jacob claimed that his family was very close and constantly worried about him, no one visited. Jacob also minimized his illness, calling it a lung condition of some sort. Many people have it much worse, but Jacob couldn't say how or what. At any rate, he asserted that the doctor promised him full recovery within 30 days because they were using very strong radiation.
>
> During the follow-up period, Jacob reported a string of symptoms, but then said that it was lack of exercise that brought on fatigue and breathlessness. His optimism was unshaken: "If the x-ray is negative, I'm cured. If it

isn't, then I'll get more treatment. I can't lose." Why hadn't anyone come with him to the clinic? "Conversation bores me. I don't like to be with people. They wanted to come but I said No!" On another occasion, he volunteered, "Worry does nobody any good, so why worry?"

After Jacob died, many months later, the social worker called on his wife and sons. They had no idea why Jacob had been going back and forth from the hospital so often, and presumably had little notion about how sick he was, even though he died at home. Stranger still was a call from a previously un-mentioned third son, who turned out to be a successful architect, unlike his indigent brothers. With a certain degree of embarrassment, he admitted that he had not kept in touch with his parents for months, perhaps years. They were both alcoholics, as were his brothers, and he had become disgusted with them all. He had not known about Jacob's death until after it happened.

PREDICTING DISTRESS

The vulnerable patient is like someone short of cash, with a small bank account, reduced income, and very little credit. Emotional and economic marginality have much in common. Those with the most resources need it least.

Who are the most vulnerable cancer patients? Can they be identified early? If high emotional distress can be compared to a fever, then some cancer patients from the outset are very sick, while others are only tempo-rarily out of sorts. Most patients are in-between, ranging from mild dismay to emotional disturbances found among psychiatric outpatients.

Extreme physical illness, especially pain, combined with drastic surgi-cal procedures, would distress practically anyone. However, psychosocial problems are not automatically created at the time of cancer diagnosis. Some physicians claim that by relieving all physical symptoms, psychoso-cial problems will soon recede. Others believe that almost every cancer patient needs counseling. Neither is correct. It is wrong to suppose that every cancer patient is equally vulnerable or at the same risk for future distress. To assert that physical treatment (or its cessation) will relieve all other problems simply relieves the physician from making a careful psycho-social appraisal.

Cancer can create or aggravate, but not eradicate problems. Table 3 contrasts psychosocial characteristics of new cancer patients who were found to have higher emotional distress (HED) and lower emotional dis-tress (LED) at the time of initial diagnosis and at intervals up to 6 months after completing treatment. Generally, HED patients were more pessimistic at the start. They had regrets about the past, and expected little or no support from family or friends, if, indeed, the latter existed. Marital prob-lems were long-standing, along with other kinds of conflicts and discon-tents. They came from lower socioeconomic strata, with marginal resources. On testing, ego strength was low, but anxiety was high.

Table 3   Correlates of Vulnerability

Higher emotional stress (HED)	Lower emotional stress (LED)
1 Pessimistic, including outcome of illness	1 Optimistic attitudes in general
2 Regrets about past	2 Fewer regrets, if any
3 History of psychiatric treatment or suicidal ideation	3 Less extensive psychiatric treatment, if any
4 High anxiety; low ego strength (MMPI)*	4 Low anxiety; high ego strength
5 Marital problems prior to cancer	5 Few marital problems, if any
6 Lower socioeconomic status	6 Higher socioeconomic status
7 More alcohol abuse	7 Abstinence or use, not abuse
8 Multiproblem background	8 Few problems in background
9 Little or no church attendance	9 Church attendance
10 More physical symptoms	10 Fewer physical symptoms
11 Cancer at advanced stage	11 Less advanced cancer stage
12 Expects little support from others	12 Expects adequate support
13 Doctor seen as less helpful	13 Doctor's help is adequate at least
14 More current concerns of all kinds	14 Fewer current concerns
15 Feels more like giving up	15 Fewer giving up feelings
16 Poor problem resolution	16 Better problem resolution
17 More Cope 4, 8, 12, 13, 15	17 More Cope 6, 7, 14
Not significant: age, marital status, lagtime until diagnosis, life stress events (Holmes-Rahe).	

*Minnesota Multiphasic Personality Inventory.

LED patients coped better, confronting, redefining, and adhering to the treatment schedule. Relationships with family and friends were good, as was their relation with the doctor. The latter is especially important because a physician who at least *asks* about nonphysical concerns may help to prevent them. Hope and concern are both contagious, and a dismal, impatient manner confirms a dejected patient's expectations while aggravating isolation and vulnerability. Earlier psychiatric problems, including a multiproblem family of origin, are likely to produce later emotional distress, if cancer develops. In short, the future repeats the past for both HED and LED patients.

Predicting psychosocial distress is not crystal gazing. It is analogous to clinical prognosis, but uses personality and physical data. One hundred percent accuracy is not expected, because everyone is vulnerable to something, including the unexpected. If survival on a significant level, decreased symptoms, and high self-esteem are among the signs of good coping and lower vulnerability, then cancer patients with a past that includes other serious sicknesses, economic marginality, failure at work, marital problems or living alone, isolation, pessimism, concomitant problems, and lower ego strength are at greater risk for the future (see Table 4). Cancer may be as unmanageable as earlier problems, so that distress accumulates as time goes on.

THE ULTIMATE DISTRESS: SUICIDE

Altruistic suicide, self-destruction for a noble cause, is almost unheard of in our culture.[5] Suicide is, I suppose, a way of coping; but from another viewpoint, it bears witness to utter hopelessness and helplessness, epitomizing suffering and waste. Contemplating suicide, however, is a form of considering alternatives, and may provide just enough consolation to get through the day or night. About 10 percent of newly diagnosed cancer patients admit to such suicidal thoughts. Actual attempts are very rare, despite widespread misconceptions to the contrary. Suicidal people are generally hopeless at the time. But not all hopeless people, or even the majority, ever become suicidal. It is like being very angry or having homicidal ideas. Considering the vast number of irate, outraged people, murder is fairly infrequent.

The relation of coping, cancer, and suicide remains an intriguing problem.[6] There are tumor experts who have never known any cancer patient who attempted suicide; some physicians with extensive experience in oncology assert that suicide attempts are less common than in the population at large. Nevertheless, the specter of potential suicide is constantly held up as

Table 4   High-Risk Patient Profile (Those Experiencing the Most Distress)

Personality:	Low ego strength, high anxiety (MMPI)
	Pessimistic
Past history:	Marital problems, if married
	Living alone
	Lower socioeconomic status
	Alcohol abuse
	Infrequent church attendance
	Multiproblem family of origin
	Psychiatric treatment
	Suicidal ideation at times
Physical status:	Advanced staging
	More reported symptoms
Plight:	More problems of all types
	Expects and receives little help
	Sees physicians as less helpful or concerned
Performance:	Cope 4 (suppression and passivity)
	Cope 8 (fatalistic submission)
	Cope 12 (isolation/withdrawal)
	Cope 13 (blame others)
	Cope 15 (blame self)
	Feels more like giving up
	Poorer resolutions

a warning and as a rationalization for not telling a patient about cancer. This contention is difficult to support.

Some patients—a very few—do attempt suicide, but seldom because of cancer.[7] Most frequently, attempts occur because of a threatened break in personal relationships, or as a protest against destructive emotions. Lonely, isolated, resentful people do become hopeless and hostile. Cancer confers no protection against suicide. But there is no convincing evidence that cancer drastically reduces the threshold to suicide. In the cases I know about, the attempt, whether completed or not, occurred just as often during remission and with tumors of low malignancy as it did with patients suffering from severe symptoms and disabilities.

Case 27 Ingrid was only 32 years old when she was found to have metastatic carcinoma of the ovary. Surgery was out of the question. Chemotherapy made her very sick. Her hair fell out; she vomited, staggered, developed ulcerations and anemia. As the disease progressed, she became more helpless. Losing control of bodily functions made her feel angry, depressed, and even insulted. Soiling herself was more than just incontinence; it was a humiliating and degrading affront. Her pain required large amounts of sedatives, which also created the problem of clouded consciousness and stupor. Being a self-reliant, immaculate, and intellectual person, her inability to converse intelligently was almost as painful and distressing as incontinence.

When I first spoke with her, Ingrid talked openly about suicide. She had no specific plans, however, and until the cancer developed, with its accompanying symptoms and disabilities, never considered self-destruction. Now it seemed about the only option left, since she had little confidence in chemotherapy or other medical procedures. Death had no inherent dread for her. What she feared most was unabating pain, as well as other kinds of suffering. I told her that the severity of the pain could almost certainly be controlled, despite our inability to slow the advance of her underlying disease. Then she asked the ultimate existential question that almost every physician fears: If the pain was not relieved, could she ask for enough medication to hasten death?

I knew she meant it. I also knew that some people are suicidal for brief periods, and then, for unknown reasons, decide to continue living, although circumstances have not changed. I could not, at that moment, promise to help her terminate the dying process, nor could I engage in platitudes designed to make her feel guilty and nonsuicidal. I merely repeated and promised that pain could be controlled, without answering her question.

She was properly dubious, but suddenly became less depressed, and began to talk about other things, including doubts about her husband's emotional stability. She had no children, having preferred freedom to pursue her career, unencumbered. Nevertheless, I was aware that incontinence, invalidism, humiliation, and pain might still lead to suicide.

During the next 6 months, I saw Ingrid from time to time, regularly when she returned to the hospital, intermittently when she was at home. Pain was not relieved, unless she took massive amounts of medication. Her family doctor permitted her to regulate the dosage by leaving a bottle of pills at her bedside.

I knew the "risk" and perhaps understood his message, and left the bottle where it was. However, despite the pain, she preferred not to interfere with mental clarity by overdosing herself into stupor. Protracted vegetation was another fear that she allayed by paying a price in pain. Remission was a vain hope. She worsened day by day. I wondered when she would remind me about helping her terminate, just as I knew that death was literally within reach. Instead, she grasped at fragile signs of encouragement, enjoying our visits, seemingly, but resenting the intrusion of erstwhile friends. Her husband fluctuated in tolerance of distress, but fortunately, a very capable nurse's aide was brought in who relieved him of many distasteful chores.

Two weeks before death, Ingrid was readmitted to the hospital for "further evaluation," a euphemism for awaiting death under medical observation. Pain was somewhat less; at least that promise had been fulfilled. She had many periods of clarity, but at no time did she mention suicide or euthanasia. Each morning, she was there, with every pill accounted for. Finally, an infection supervened, and at last, she died.

Ingrid was not afraid of dying, only of pain and further humiliation. Nevertheless, with every opportunity to overdose, and no questions asked, she did not. One night, stuporous with pain and pills, she forgot how much medication she had taken. In alarm, she rang for the nurse. The following morning she told me about the episode, saying, "I guess the will to live must still be pretty strong."

Ingrid's plight emphasizes a fact that is more significant than a disposition towards suicide. The plight of having cancer, even terminal cancer, with all its suffering and disability, may underscore the value of life enough that it is not easily thrown away. Committing suicide may be an ultimate option, but it violates or usurps the values held most precious during active life. It appropriates death, and reminds us that even unequivocally suicidal patients frequently expect to survive in some strange, qualified way, freed of the turmoil that left them no other course.[8] Generally, even the most hopeless dejected cancer patient lacks the sadistic, self-punitive drive of suicidal patients seen by psychiatrists. Nevertheless, because existential despair is at the core of vulnerability, I ask very distressed cancer patients about suicidal thoughts in the recent past, especially when they mention hopelessness. Those few cancer patients who have attempted suicide, even before the diagnosis, usually are driven to this extremity by family strife, alcoholism, or paranoid hatred of others. Hopelessness about cancer is never offered as a sufficient reason. There are, I believe, many other patients like Ingrid who simply consider suicide as an ultimate response to unbearable distress, but in whom the fires of life still burn.

REFERENCES

1 Greer, H., "Psychological Correlates of Breast Cancer," in B. Stoll (ed.), *Risk Factors in Breast Cancer,* William Heinemann Medical Books, Chicago, 1976, chap. 5, pp. 70–79.

2 Hillman, J., *Emotion: A Comprehensive Phenomenology of Theories and Their Meanings for Therapy,* Routledge & Kegan Paul, Ltd., London, 1960.
3 Wessman, A., and D. Ricks, *Mood and Personality,* Holt, Rinehart and Winston, Inc., New York, 1966.
4 Janis, I., *Psychological Stress: Psychoanalytic and Behavioral Studies of Surgical Patients,* John Wiley & Sons, Inc., New York, 1958.
5 Maris, R., *Social Forces in Urban Suicide,* The Dorsey Press, Homewood, Ill., 1969, chap. 2, "Durkheim's Theory of Suicide," pp. 20–44.
6 Weisman, A., "Coping Behavior and Suicide in Cancer," in *Cancer: The Behavioral Dimensions,* J. Cullen, B. Fox, and R. Isom (eds.), Raven Press, New York, 1976, pp. 331–341.
7 Farberow, N., S. Ganzler, F. Cutter, and D. Reynolds, "An Eight-Year Survey of Hospital Suicides," *Life-threatening Behavior,* **1**: 184–202, 1971.
8 Weisman, A., "Is Suicide a Disease?" *Life-threatening Behavior,* **1**(4): 219–231, 1971.

Seven Areas of Concern

WHAT DO CANCER PATIENTS WORRY ABOUT?

If a tear were shed for every problem and moment of despair endured by people, the oceans of the world would surely overflow and engulf us all. Cancer patients are concerned about everything other people face, besides the uncertainty and chronicity of illness. After a diagnosis of cancer, the spreading network of distress makes any distinction between cancer-related problems and fortuitous events somewhat academic.

Even before an illness can be called a disease, psychosocial equilibrium may be shaky. Physicians sometimes forget that patients are sick, and that hospital admission for the individual is an important event. Consequently, once in the hospital, a person runs a risk of becoming another number. Previous circumstances are somewhat irrelevant, although very "important" people usually carry their prominence with them, like a banner. For the most part, however, personal problems and pressing concerns become peripheral, at best. Silence covers earlier distress and, like a veil, obscures problems that lie ahead. Problems are private.

While their number is astronomical, problems and concerns overlap so much that counting and classification, even naming, are inadequate and provisional. But then, the famous seven warning signals of cancer, such as changes in bowel habits, discoloration of a mole, unexplained lumps, and so forth, are themselves only signposts. They are not diagnostic of cancer, nor do they cover the full range of clinical manifestations by which cancer can announce itself. Similarly, there is nothing absolute about the seven areas of concern to be described in this chapter (see Table 5). They are really domains in which individual problems can and do occur, like seven continents with many countries, large and small, whose names, prominence, and boundaries are always changing.

Each area of concern can implicate other domains, again demonstrating their permeability. For example, one day a woman receiving radiation for breast cancer reported that her son had fallen from a tree, broken his arm, and missed school for several days. Upsetting to her, of course, but to the doctor, the episode, if he listened at all, had no connection with her illness and treatment. However, as a result of radiation treatment, she felt very fatigued and depleted. She did housework, cooked meals, and so forth, but was otherwise unable to resume her regular life. In fact, she privately considered herself to be utterly inept, inadequate, and inconsequential.

That radiation could itself cause fatigue meant nothing to her. In her eyes, she was not just fatigued; she was weak, indifferent, and negligent. Her son's fall and fracture, therefore, were not unrelated to cancer. "I wasn't around. I should have kept my eye on him, so that he wouldn't take chances like that. But I can't do anything, or not much. I've already failed my husband, now my son. What's going to happen next?"

CONCERNS AND PROBLEMS

Tillich considered religion the ultimate concern.[1] I believe that the quest for survival, security, sustenance, and significance is not only our basic concern, but that there are many styles, avenues, and methods by which we can reach these goals. Reaching out is itself a matter of continuous coping, because fulfillment is apt to be very temporary, soon overtaken by new problems.

Table 5   Areas of Predominant Concern

Health
Self-appraisal
Work and finances
Family and significant relationships
Religion
Friends and associates
Existential

Concerns and problems are related, but different issues. A *concern* is anything one worries about. A *problem*, however, is a task yet to be done, a question to be answered, a quandary to be solved, an enigma to be clarified. If not dealt with, we become distressed. A concern belongs to the here-and-now. A problem is an obstacle to the future, arising out of present concerns. When a cancer patient is first evaluated, therefore, it is proper to ask questions, such as, "What are some of the problems you now see yourself facing?" or, "What are you mainly concerned about?" Part of a physician's job is to identify concomitant problems that might impede treatment, convalescence, or recovery. If a physician cannot do this, then he is, at the most, competent but limited. He is disengaged from the person who happens to be his patient. But if he elucidates pressing concerns, he promotes the coping process.

Pious admonitions to consider the "patient as a whole" are inadequate for this task. More is required than simply uttering convenient platitudes about "support," "courage," "time will tell," and so forth. Nevertheless, just a question put at the right time to a concerned patient may make an incredible difference. Merely asking, "How has this illness changed you or your life?" signifies that the doctor cares, shares, and fortifies. His comments may even reduce vulnerability.

Squaring the circle of illness depends upon the nature of disease, adequate coping, reduced vulnerability, and minimal problems. Together, they combine forces to produce psychosocial effectiveness. At the outset, a physician assigns or attributes physical symptoms to one organ system or another, but ultimately every symptom interacts. The same is true for areas of concern.

Most of the specific problems which vex cancer patients, or anyone else, fall within the domains of health, self-appraisal, work and finances, family and significant relationships, religion, friends and associates, and existential concerns. Other categories are certainly feasible, and the reader is invited to make up different alignments.[2]

Health Concerns　Almost every patient wants to get better, but getting better, especially from chronic illness, has a wider scope than just losing symptoms. Basically, it refers to health delivery, continuity of care, effects of treatment, medical costs, ancillary physical problems, and so forth. Many health considerations appear unrelated to what a doctor considers the primary goal of curing cancer. But health concerns are persistent, and sometimes patients do not know how or when to speak about them.

> "My sleep is very disturbed. I seldom get to sleep before 3 or 4 A.M., and then dream so much. I hate to bother Dr. R., because he's so busy, and the main thing is to take treatment."

"The shots make me sick all over. I get a funny taste in my mouth. No one ever told me about that, so I guess it isn't very important. The cancer needs to be knocked out, once and for all. So I'm not complaining."

"I only get the runaround here. Why bother asking? If the doctor had anything to say, he'd say it. If he cared at all, he'd ask me. I'm getting fed up."

"I can't pay for all this medicine. Is it okay to take half as much and make it last twice as long?"

"I paid good money into the union all these years. Now they say they can't pay for my treatment. That's happening with everything, it seems."

"I feel better than ever. Why do I have to keep coming back? Do they think I can get sick again?"

"My doctor is really great. She says the tumor seems to be shrinking, but that it is still too early to tell."

"How can I get well when these shots and pills only make me sicker? The doctor ought to know that!"

Self-appraisal Concerns   Not only does almost every patient want to get better, but to survive, and survive well. Standards depend on self-esteem, proficiency, approval of others, images of what one might have done or become, recollections of competence, significance, and general feelings of how one fits into the scheme of objects, people, and things that matter most. Self-appraisal can be dimmed by pessimism, past regrets, and failures. Overly high expectations, likewise, can void and distort self-evaluation. Few people are so self-sufficient that their attitude is not mirrored and influenced by the assumed attitude of others. Consequently, a cancer patient is not only confronted with potential or actual physical changes, but with what might happen to self-concept, goals, appearance, disability, functions, and security in an uncertain future.

"I sometimes think people treat me too well, at least they seem so different, compared with how they used to be. Everyone is kind, almost too kind. I don't need such kindness. Just treat me as I was before. I make people uncomfortable. Maybe it's because they're not sick. But actually I don't feel sick. I think it's because they haven't had cancer and don't know what it's like, and I do."

"I'm not the same in any way. I just don't feel at home in my body. Does that sound funny? I keep saying that I shouldn't do this or that. It's really because I can't do them anyway, and it makes me feel better to pretend that I don't want to do them!"

"I used to enjoy getting out on the beach. Now I'm ashamed to have anyone see me, stare at me with this big scar."

"I get tired out. If my body is so weak, I wonder if my mind is slipping, too."

"The kids used to jump in bed with me every morning. Now they're very careful, and look at me funny."

"I hate being me!"

"I get so irritable. It's surprising that I don't fly out or up or whatever you call it, at anyone coming near me, even you!"

"Since the treatment, my doctor told me not to get excited and be calm. So I get depressed."

Work and Financial Concerns It requires no special insight to understand that when the breadwinner is ill, income often ceases, savings vanish, sick leave runs out, insurance is inadequate, and chronic unemployment becomes a way of life. Few families can withstand the drain and strain of prolonged and catastrophic illness.[3] Public assistance may be needed, and much more.

In our society, the ruling ethic is that to be workless is to be worthless. Job or occupation are not just sources of income, but of personal worth and well-being. Cancer patients who are forced to leave their jobs lack the rationalization that it is an act of choice. Even for the fortunate few who do have enough money, status, and security, the idea of being on the shelf, unemployable, or half-employed is a distressing, if not humiliating, experience, far greater than fear of death. Boredom and obsolescence are two benign complications. Other self-appraisal afflictions are more devastating.

"I don't know how I can afford such lengthy treatment. My wife is willing to go back to work, but she hasn't taught school for over 25 years. Jobs are scarce. Here I am, after all these years, counting pennies!"

"If I had a steady income, I could get better treatment. Sitting here in the clinic reminds me that I'm just a number. I feel like a parasite, regardless that it isn't my fault. I never wanted to be a burden, but if you ain't got the dough, who are you?"

"I'm still working. How long they'll put up with me is something else. My boss knows I can only work so long. He probably thinks I'm not doing a good job, and I'm not!"

"I have plenty of money to live on. I was almost ready to retire anyway. But I feel like an extra wheel when I look out the window and see everyone going to work in the morning. Sometimes I wish I could leave the house, and pretend I had an office to go to!"

Family and Significant Relationships Families are the stuff of intimacy, satisfaction, hopes, fears, and misery. Few cancer patients embark on their new life without an impact on their families or significant others, who substitute for families. Patients who expect little or no support are usually correct, either through choice, collusion, or circumstances. There are many widows in this plight. Married in an era when women were solely expected to be homemakers, they find themselves utterly alone, lonely, living on meager pensions, and without resources. Not everyone, of course, depends on family and significant others, or wants to. Self-sufficient loners rarely view their situation with much regret. But self-sufficiency has limitations. Even loners look to a problematic future in which they can no longer work or take care of themselves.

Cancer often creates embarrassing problems within the family that physicians seldom know about. Sterility, impotence, sexual inhibitions, and social restrictions are topics that many patients seemingly accept without complaint. However, regardless of the apparent resolution, sexuality and child-rearing are never to be taken for granted. A patient needs to discuss relevant sexual matters, regardless of marital status.

Sexuality is, however, but one element of family interaction. Intimacy and mutual regard are even more important. "What's been the effect on your family?" is a straightforward question that needs asking for a candid answer. Families are not always the staunchest ally, and it is a mistake to assume that any patient relies most on those who are officially related by birth or marriage. Attitudes to people cover much more than deep affection, quivering ambivalence, or cold indifference. Who are the *significant key others* in anyone's life?

> "Old Dad can't earn a living any more. Yes, I hate to admit it, but I do wonder how the kids will treat me, now that the pump is broken and the well is almost dry."

> "I hate to ask anyone for anything, Doctor. Especially my brothers. You might say that they've been more successful than me. Always been that way since we were boys. When they drive up in their big cars, I just wilt and want to shrink up. I'd rather rot than let on that I need anything!"

> "My wife used to depend on me. Now it's the other way round."

> "I always intended to leave my wife, but kept putting it off. Now I'd like to get some fun out of life, whatever that is."

> "You know, this cancer has brought us all closer together, like we're starting over. That's a funny thought, but time seems to mean less and more, even little things."

> "My daughter has always been a very good girl. She would never go out on a date without first getting my approval. No, she never married, but she works hard. I still count on her, especially since my husband died. We have no one else."

> "My daughter just thinks about herself. No job, dates every night till all hours. Never tells me anything, even when I bawl her out. I never had it so good. My mother died when I was 16, and I never had a chance at education. But my husband takes her side, she can just twist him around her finger."

"I live alone, and want to keep it that way. No, I don't want my parents to know I'm sick."

"My wife is all I have. I just look at her, sitting there day after day. What will her life be like after I'm gone?"

Religion   Even in an increasingly secular world, religious affiliations and institutions are still strong, holding vast numbers of people together in mutual creeds and needs. For many, religion is the only link with transcendental ideas, and churches are the major focus of community relationships. Belief in an afterlife does not seem to change human behavior, nor do transmundane values mollify the fear of death.[4] However, church membership and attendance do offer group cohesion and, very often, mutual consolation at times of grief.

Some patients feel remiss about not attending church regularly, and promise to mend their ways. These resolutions are usually short-lived, scarcely outlasting the initial impact of cancer. But for regular churchgoers, it is the place to make and keep friends, find approval, and seek guidance.

Many patients are not only agnostic, but find religious ideas to be anathema. They do not seem to suffer, and often cope very well. Nevertheless, for others, the clergy is a strong ally, providing pastoral care, counseling, and continuity after hospital discharge. But the influence of theological concepts on coping competence is another matter which is difficult to assess.

Church attenders do seem to have lower levels of distress. From one viewpoint, this would prove that belief in God is a good thing. From another viewpoint, lower vulnerability among church attenders merely shows that church is an excellent conduit for human relationships, especially for those who depend on more conventional support systems. Furthermore, members of the clergy are likely to be compassionate men and women who care about people, even more than they care about official beliefs and credos. They listen well, attend to details in relationships, and do not sacrifice the individual to ritualistic requirements.

We are, I suppose, all fellow pilgrims on this earth.[5] Theological beliefs are not obligatory in order to think about basic issues of life, death, and destiny. Church attendance does not automatically mean that a person is deeply devout. Nevertheless, very sick cancer patients will often muse about theology in some form, or have it suggested to them by visitors and friends.

"I wish I could feel closer to God."

"I lost my early religious faith, and now I wish I hadn't."

"I'd feel like a hypocrite if I even considered any help from religion. It's okay for those who are sold on it."

"Yes, I think about life and death, what it would be like to see old friends again. But right now, talking about friends, I'm just worried about moving out of my old neighborhood."

"I don't go to church. Too many phonies there. But I believe in prayer, even if I don't pray very much."

"When you're sick, I say, why not try anything?"

"If I really believed in God, I'd ask what this cancer is all about!"

Friends and Associates   At times of crisis or illness, friends come in handy, regardless of personal independence. But most friendships are circumscribed in time, depth, intimacy, and commitment. Friends and associates do tend to rally round the sick bed, but not for very long or very much, which is the way it is supposed to be. After a while, patients cease looking for support from friends, accepting what is offered, knowing that people are usually uncomfortable in sickrooms.

There is a ceiling and a season for most relationships. Naturally, it is reassuring to have someone to count on, but counting on someone means that the other person fills a specific function, like a doctor or minister, and is not expected to be useful in any other capacity. Newly diagnosed patients do not rank friends and associates very high with respect to problems and concerns. This does not diminish the value of friendship, but rather signifies limited expectations and that other concerns are more pressing.

"I heard about a man with cancer who had to quit his job because the other guys thought it was contagious. Hardly anyone spoke to him, wouldn't even eat with him. What kind of way is that to treat anyone?"

"Sure, I have lots of friends. They've told me just to call if I need anything. I don't happen to need anything, that's all, so I don't see much of them."

"The women at my office are great! They're more like sisters. In fact, I like them better than my sister."

"Friends? Sure, the bar is full of them every night!"

Existential Concerns   Regardless of how persistently physicians and cancer societies "accentuate the positive" and reassure the public at large, cancer is still bonded to the grim notion of uncertainty and terminality, as if no one ever died of anything else. Vulnerability originates in existential despair, but not every patient can verbalize its shadowy implications and intimations. Some people think about death very often, while others, hardly ever. Nevertheless, existential concerns are not at all confined to the ruminations of a few philosophers and theologians. They are inherent to most human problems.[6]

I am committed to the viewpoint that the fabric of life is interwoven with threads of death, but that thoughts of death and finitude, instead of being morbid, put a fine edge on the here-and-now of existence. In clinical work with cancer patients, existential concerns are probably uppermost, but still hidden. Consequently, one must glean thoughts about life and death from seemingly random remarks. For example, a comment, "I wish my children were settled in life," expresses a family problem, but it is also a worry about not being around to see children grow up.

"Will I live or die? Of course, sometime, but not now!"

"How much life can anyone be sure of? Even funeral directors and doctors die, too, you know."

"Night school takes so much time. Maybe I ought to enjoy free time with my wife and kids, without worrying so much or sweating over some textbook."

"I look at my kids and wonder what they'll be like when they grow up."

"If life is like an elevator, I sure as hell am in the subbasement!"

"I go into a bar, have a drink, but I can't laugh it up the way I used to. Guys talk to me, but . . . I can't. . . . Shit, Doctor, what's it all about?"

CRITICAL PERIODS

For at least 70 percent of new cancer patients, the first 2 to 3 months are the most distressing. After that, problems tend to settle down, except for periodic exacerbations related to treatments, recurrences, and unexpected events. Counting concerns is not a sufficient method for determining the degree of distress. Certain problems snowball, persist, and pyramid as time goes on.

Regardless of site, stage, type of cancer, or time of assessment, practically every patient ranks existential, work, self-appraisal, and health concerns over religion, family, and friends. While work and family problems arise very early, i.e., at diagnosis, with the passage of time, family concerns tend to diminish. At critical moments, which come at any time, existential and self-appraisal concerns always predominate, as if we are abruptly prodded into thinking about who we are and where we are going.

Family problems abate, not because a patient is really less concerned, but because other issues are more intrusive. For example, a father of young children, initially concerned about working and supporting his family, sooner or later realizes that he will not go back to work and that other sources of support must be sought. Consequently, in later reviewing his plight, he will probably voice worries in terms of life and death (existential) and self-image (self-appraisal).

Patients readily relinquish medical care to physicians. Self-appraisal and existential concerns, however, persist and permeate everything else. Moreover, unsettled psychosocial problems can propagate themselves, causing as much exasperation and futility as the most disabling physical symptoms.

Case 28   Helen and Fred personified all the traditional values of middle-class America. They lived in a small New England town, where their four sons were born. Fred was an engineer, and Helen, evidently, was a contented mother and wife.

Everything went smoothly until Fred's company merged with a conglomerate. He lost his job. About a year later, Helen developed breast cancer. At the time of surgery, 20 to 22 nodes were affected. The outlook was poor.-

Fred could find only temporary work. Family finances were very low. Then Fred's widowed mother had a heart attack, and moved in with the struggling family. The oldest son joined a bizarre religious cult. He disowned his parents because they were not "true believers," but he did not leave home until he told Helen that she developed cancer because of "hatred inside." The second son became hooked on hard street drugs, dropped out of school, and the third son was in a serious automobile accident. The accident not only put further strain on the family's budget, but wrecked the old car that Fred used for intermittent jobs. For some reason, the youngest son stayed in school, pursuing ordinary life without any remarkable problems.

Meanwhile, all was not well with Helen. Her mastectomy caused severe arm pain and swelling. There were also vertebral metastases and incessant back pain. Walking was painful and difficult. Housework, cooking, and so forth were almost impossible, without extraordinary effort. "Be careful," Fred once cautioned, "you're not supposed to walk so much." She snapped, "No, and I'm not supposed to have cancer, either!" While she was understandably reluctant to ask questions about the extent of cancer, she explained that her neck hurt because of slipping on the ice, months before. Nevertheless, she felt demoralized, angry, and useless. She would rave about nothing in particular, frequently blaming Fred because he was the only one handy.

Helen lived for another 18 months. Her major concern was what would happen to her sons and husband "if I should die." She also requested a strict Catholic funeral, although she had not attended church for years. About 6 months before death, Helen was readmitted, weak and cachectic. She wondered how she ever thought that this thing (i.e., cancer) could be fought, yearning for earlier days when "I was still a person." One day she reported that Fred had finally found a regular job (possibly true) and that her oldest son had telephoned, wishing her a speedy recovery (probably false). After her death, Fred called the social worker, asking for advice about raising his two younger sons, who remained at home. But when the worker later tried to call, the phone had been disconnected. He left no forwarding address.

I cite this case mainly because in it every domain of concern is represented. That cancer constitutes a personal challenge as well as a psychosocial calamity needs no further documentation. However, as this tragedy unfolded during Helen's sickness, doctors were hardly aware of it. Whether these multiple misfortunes could be attached to the medical plight is rather irrelevant. What is sure, however, is that just as vulnerability rises and falls, problems and concerns ebb and flow, like waves amid the tides. Only a few people are totally engulfed, but storms can affect anyone during critical periods. When this happens, refuge is needed. Alienation and apprehension pass back and forth through physical distress and psychosocial problems. It is not astonishing to find that distressing problems early in the course of cancer are like clouds gathering on the horizon, signifying a storm ahead.

Prudent physicians and devoted families should be aware of critical periods in order to introduce countercoping strategies which shelter, or at least ameliorate, the future. No one can be assured of complete correction of every problem, nor can professionals of any persuasion or competence benefit everyone. But partial benefits are better than none. Cancerology, of all specialties, should appreciate limitations inherent to psychosocial interventions. Overwhelming success in abolishing problems is a rare reward. Coping with cancer is accustomed to limited goals.

REFERENCES

1   Tillich, P., *The Eternal Now,* Charles Scribner's Sons, New York, 1963.
2   Duff, R., and A. Hollingshead, *Sickness and Society,* Harper & Row Publishers, Incorporated, New York, Evanston, and London, 1968.
3   Pollack, J., "Observations on the Economics of Illness," in *Catastrophic Illness in the Seventies: Critical Issues and Complex Decisions,* Fourth Annual Symposium, Cancer Care, Inc., of the National Cancer Foundation, New York, 1970, pp. 20–32.
4   Feifel, H., "Religious Conviction and Fear of Death among the Healthy and Terminally Ill," *Journal for the Scientific Study of Religion,* **13**:3 (September 1974), 353–360.
5   Hiltner, S., *Pastoral Counseling,* Abingdon Press, Nashville and New York, 1949.
6   Shneidman, E., *Deaths of Man,* Quadrangle/New York Times Book Co., New York, 1973.

Psychosocial Staging in Cancer

THE CONCEPT OF STAGING

Most cancer specialists agree that *cancer* is a term that is almost too inclusive, considering how many tumors and malignant processes have been identified. Classification of cancer is largely based on anatomical and microscopic (histological) observations. Its purpose is to account for all possible presentations of cancer in and around organ systems. The purpose of cancer *staging,* however, is to define the actual extent of cancer when it is first diagnosed, because treatment is evaluated according to the stage of the tumor or malignant process at the time of diagnosis. The most common mode of staging is based on tumor, nodes, and metastases, called the TNM system.[1] However, despite constant refinement, clinicians are generally dissatisfied with the TNM method because few cancers follow a neat three-stage progression. Moreover, depth of invasiveness may be a better criterion for cancer staging than size, spread, or dissemination. The staging system, as it now stands, has tended to branch out more and more, so that with new information, staging for one organ cannot be compared precisely with staging for another. There are too many exceptions and loopholes. In fact, Terry, a pathologist, states that tumors are as unique as the patients in whom they occur.[2]

Staging a tumor is an active process—in the mind of the oncologist. Clinicians tend to use very private assessments, or make valiant attempts to find a standard scheme. Each organ system seems to have its special problems, which defy the TNM model. Nevertheless, staging helps a physician plan and evaluate treatment, prognosticate, and learn more about whatever is being staged. Generally, the following system has been recommended, and widely adopted in principle:[3]

Stage 1   Disease limited to the organ in which it originated
Stage 2   Disease located just outside the primary organ, with no other organ involvement or lymph node metastasis
Stage 3   Disease that has spread to regional lymph nodes
Stage 4   Disease that involves distant organs and remote nodes

Some years ago, Feinstein observed that systems for staging cancer were predominantly anatomical, that is, based on shape, structure, and spread, and that concomitant clinical status was not considered.[4] In trying to overcome this ambiguity, i.e., calling an anatomical system "clinical," Feinstein made many other contributions to clinical epidemiology.

For my purposes, however, Feinstein's most important suggestion was to combine clinical status with anatomical staging, which, as I have indicated, depends more upon invasiveness than on TNM.[5a,5b] He first reduced anatomical stages from four to three:

1   Localized tumors
2   Regionally invasive tumors
3   Distantly disseminated tumors

Then he arranged patients clinically:

1   Patients without symptoms or with primary symptoms of long duration
2   Patients with systemic symptoms or with primary symptoms of short duration
3   Patients with symptoms of metastatic dissemination

Stage 1 was called *Indolent;* stage 2, *Obtrusive;* stage 3, *Deleterious.*

Having assigned patients to 9 groups (3 $\times$ 3), combining clinical and anatomical factors, Feinstein proposed four new, clinicoanatomical stages, A, B, C, and D. These correlated well, it turned out, with survival rates. That is, each stage was an aggregate of patients with comparable prognoses, a factor not directly related to anatomy.

The details and further development of this concept need not be reported here. From the psychosocial standpoint, the essential issue is that anatomy is not everything, even in cancer. Clinical status, symptoms, and prognosis differ in patients with similar histological lesions and distribution. One patient may not be greatly disabled until distant lesions and deleterious symptoms develop. Another patient, with an identical cancer, may be very sick or die far earlier. This finding provides me with a precedent for the observation that cancer patients at the same stage may also differ widely in their capacity to cope, endure problems, and maintain a low level of vulnerability.

PSYCHOSOCIAL STAGING

The psychosocial dimension of cancer is incontrovertible. However, I propose to amplify clinical and anatomical staging by adding a series of psychosocial stages. Perhaps psychosocial factors at different stages also contribute to the expected survival of certain cancer patients.[6]

A proposal of this kind is not without other precedents. For example, people do not age or even learn at the same pace or in the same way. Growing older is a process which may be indolent, obtrusive, or deleterious. Chronological age is a conceptual convenience, not much more. It helps demographers measure age along a continuum for special purposes, using different parameters. Sooner or later, effects of aging may spread to all parts of the mind and body, inducing senility, severe arteriosclerosis, and other impairments. Meanwhile, some men, aged 75, will seem or be physiologically and mentally younger than other men of the same age. Psychosocial assets or coping capacity may even contribute to slowing down of the aging process.[7]

Therefore, I postulate four psychosocial stages, which may be considered in conjunction with, if not parallel to, four clinicoanatomical stages:

1 Existential plight
2 Mitigation and accommodation
3 Decline and deterioration
4 Preterminality and terminality

Stages 3 and 4 can be combined into early and late phases. This concept of staging is based on psychosocial effectiveness, just as physical staging is based on invasiveness, spread, cellular differentiation, and so forth.

Stage 1: Existential Plight

Theoretically, the medical plight should begin in the prediagnostic period, when signs that something is awry first present themselves. However, conventional staging is determined at the time of diagnosis, not before. So psychosocial staging should begin at that point, too.

There are two initial substages: impact distress and existential plight proper.

Impact distress is what happens at that moment when a patient first definitely learns about cancer. Naturally, that moment is not instantaneous, but rather refers loosely to the here-and-now surrounding the diagnostic period.

Existential plight proper includes impact, but goes beyond that time to the point when primary treatment ends, when the patient attempts to resume ordinary life. Roughly, it covers the first 3 to 4 months, or, for convenience, the first 100 days or so.[8]

How distressing *is* impact distress? Even though the best treatment is given first, it is often an alarming moment. At least one-third of our research patients saw death as a real possibility, regardless of treatment, prognosis, or site. The sobering fact of family deaths from cancer still did not seem to determine the level of existential distress.

Existential plight proper is, then correctly called "Plight's Peak." While some cancer patients become more distressed as the disease progresses, nevertheless, coping well during the first 100 days or so makes it likely that a patient will continue to cope effectively. An early low vulnerability rating is usually a good sign, in spite of unforeseen peaks that may arise later.

During the early months, however, distress is likely to be proportionate to the severity of physical symptoms. Later, especially at critical periods (see Chapter 6) that fortuitously develop, psychosocial factors become more and more important. Nevertheless, the more serious the cancer at the outset, the more difficulty is experienced in subsequent adaptation. Even successful treatment of lung cancer changes a patient's life. If a bladder cancer requires complete resection, psychosocial equilibrium will definitely and instantaneously be disturbed.

Stage 2: Mitigation and Accommodation

Because cancer patients, like everyone else, cope in different ways, it is difficult to find a rubric or phrase comprehensive enough to cover properly the unfolding, diversified process of perception, performance, correction, and control which is the essence of active adaptation. Some patients do very well; others, not so well; still others manage, with effort. The psychosocial analogue of established disease, with and without clinical activity, is best called "mitigation" and "accommodation."

Psychosocial Stage 2 can last indefinitely. Its duration ranges from patients who have an early and permanent remission or cure to those who remain sick or worsen, almost as soon as primary treatment ends. For example, patients with cancer of the esophagus are in deep trouble during the existential plight. Symptoms continue; patients try to cope, seeking mitigation and accommodation, but the illness has too great a velocity.

Regardless of its duration, mitigation and accommodation are measured by distress dissipated and autonomy regained. Partial recovery or semi-invalidism may be the best result obtainable. An amputee learns to use a prosthesis and restrict certain physical activities. Chronicity does not necessarily mean invalidism. Other patients are apparently cured of cancer, but for psychosocial reasons, remain disabled and discontented. The cancer may be inactive, but so are they. A clean colostomy, for example, is consistent with a full life, but not for everyone. Side effects, such as loss of sexual powers, require family readjustment that seldom comes to the attention of physicians or nurses. Thus, regardless of physical outcome and lack of progression, there are many patients who remain subclinically vulnerable, as they attempt mitigation of and accommodation to a variety of psychosocial problems.

There is surprisingly little documentation about the quality of life in "cured" or long-surviving cancer patients. Some clinicians find that these patients may have reassessed their life, and presumably are better people for having experienced a life-threatening illness.[9] Schonfield, however, found that women with higher covert anxiety after a mastectomy were less likely to resume their precancer occupation or style of life.[10] Ten years after mastectomy, according to Schottenfeld and Robbins, there were no differences between women who had regional or localized breast cancer, followed by mastectomy.[11] Both groups had the same degree of successful rehabilitation. Obviously, women with metastatic disease at diagnosis had more difficulty in adjusting, if, indeed, they survived ten years. Cope has reminded us that radical mastectomy is not indicated for every woman with breast cancer, because some malignancies are inherently less invasive and more indolent than others.[12] Nevertheless, mastectomy, as well as other kinds of cancer surgery, imposes certain psychosocial problems that a substantial number of women find difficult to solve.[13]

Anatomical staging is apparently not the best predictor of subsequent adaptation, unless, of course, the disease is far advanced at diagnosis. Loss of morale, persistent health concerns, and painful, private preoccupations may be more significant in differentiating patients who fail to return to work or adjust in other respects. Some cancer patients find that psychosocial or economic obstacles impede their accommodation, whether or not they are physically disabled. Conversely, signs of good coping, such as optimism, capacity to correct, and reasonable assertiveness are attributes of having mitigated and accommodated to the fact of cancer, and favor a better quality of life.

Stage 3: Decline and Deterioration

The transition from psychosocial Stage 2 to decline and deterioration sometimes happens without obvious physical changes. Patients may start to lose weight, become more fatigued, irritable, anorexic, and depressed. Patients who have been living well without apparent disease suddenly slip, even without evidence of recurrence.

Naturally, recurrences require further treatment. More than one recurrence, especially when accompanied by serious physical signs, such as fever or unexplained biochemical phenomena, foreshadow the advent of still more illness and less effective treatment. At this phase, the term "palliation" is often introduced, meaning that only relief can be offered.[14]

Palliation is a word that means cloak, mask, disguise, or shroud (*pallium*). Its use is both ironic and literal, because every effort is usually made to cover up, to pretend, to disguise the prognosis, which, indeed, is shrouded. What *is* happening is that a patient has reached a point of no return, regardless of treatment. Not only does medical treatment fail to contain or restrain physical symptoms, but the intangible quality of life also deteriorates.

Stage 4: Preterminality and Terminality

Some cancer patients carry a gloomy prognosis for years, without becoming preterminal. Their decline is so slow and indolent that impairment is merely a symptom of chronicity. Preterminality, however, is not only a sign of decline and deterioration, but of accelerating irreversibility, as if decline becomes much steeper.

Decline and deterioration, therefore, have the same relation to preterminality as repeated recurrences have to progressive cachexia, fever, and severe metabolic abnormalities. The latter stage emerges from the more limited earlier stage. The important consideration is that preterminality is when dying begins. Glaser and Strauss systematically described the sociology of impending death.[15] Nevertheless, the physiology of when dying begins is less clear.[16] Persistent fevers, intoxication, infection, and so forth tend to be typical of terminality, not the earlier phase of preterminality when weight loss, anorexia, and so forth begin.[17] The phenomenon of sudden unexpected death remains to be studied.

Kübler-Ross stages of denial, anger, bargaining, depression, and acceptance are often mistakenly considered to follow each other in an inflexible sequence.[18] Literally, some people liken these stages to Stations of the Cross that every traveler must stop at before reaching final acceptance and death at some private Calvary. However, her stages are not all invariant or even typical of all dying patients, but may also occur in almost anyone who faces a serious loss or unwanted change in status, such as losing a spouse, going on welfare, or being forced to move away from a familiar neighborhood. In fact, denial is often found mixed in with anger and depression. Bargaining is very common. Acceptance comes and goes. All five stages can be found in a single interview.

As a rule, preterminal patients tend to yield active responsibility, either by asking for help, or withdrawing from further efforts to help themselves. The preterminal and terminal stage is frequently more difficult for the observer, since the patient is usually obtunded or semicomatose, as life draws to a close. Some physicians, nurses, and social workers of long experience freely admit that they never become wholly accustomed to watching someone slip slowly and inexorably toward death.

I followed a cancer patient for many months before she died, and seemed to accept her inevitable demise. Nevertheless, several weeks later, I had this dream:

> I was dressed in a surgical gown, having assisted at an operation for the patient. This puzzled me because it had been many years since I scrubbed in for surgery. A nurse then came in and told me that Mrs. X was in the recovery room, but doing well. I felt very pleased, to put it mildly.

True, I was a "surgeon's assistant" in that I had taken over psychosocial care during her waning months. But my dream made me into an actual assistant, who really helped, and did not merely preside. My patient was in the recovery room, doing well. She was not dead, and I was reassured that my efforts made a tangible contribution. Evidently, although I was relieved when Mrs. X was finally liberated from a very painful terminal illness, I still harbored an unrealistic wish that she could be operated on and then recover. Obviously, I had not wholly accepted her death.

Despite the other reservations that this dream shows, I believe that physicians, as well as others who care about the person likely to pass soon from something to nothingness, can provide safe conduct until the end. Simple presence, as contrasted with tacit retreat and withdrawal (Cope 12), can help the patient and family cope during the remaining period. Pain relief is paramount. But in some instances, narcotic needs lessen toward the end. Perhaps the body's own secretion of enkephalins contributes to somnolence and pain relief.[19] In any event, the difference between a good, bad, or equivocal death may depend upon how readily support can be asked for, mobilized, and received.

Preterminality, not terminality, is the time to effect a transition and to exchange active strategies for those that depend more on passive cooperation. The Jaffees coined the phrase "Coda syndrome," to express a final synchrony of feelings between patient and family.[20] The *Coda* is qualitatively different from actual terminality, where physiological reactions predominate and obscure the scene.

During prolonged remission or apparent cure, which I term psychosocial Stage 2 (mitigation and accommodation), a patient can reinvest in life, and even proceed as if nothing drastic has happened. During psychosocial Stage 4, and the latter phases of Stage 3, the independence that typifies good coping may be diminished. It is therefore proper to observe and encourage the exchange of active for more passive strategies during Stage 3. Then, when a patient does decline further, it is already clear what that person is most comfortable about relinquishing. Eleventh-hour heroics may add more misery than benefit, as well as confusing everyone.

Middle knowledge is a good example of how psychosocial factors, such as equivocation about treatment or giving mixed messages, can create a false optimism at a preterminal physical stage. Under very favorable circumstances, some cancer patients with advanced disease (anatomical Stage 3) can remain vigorous and productive in almost every respect, as if in psychosocial Stage 2, for a surprisingly long time. If this can be implemented more strategically, the ensuing decline and preterminality, which may be unavoidable, will be shorter and less distressing to everyone.

> *Case 29*   Mary was 52 years old, an unmarried office worker who lived with a widowed mother, but was surrounded by a large, affectionate family of brothers and sisters who were nearby. Not having a private life of her own did not seem to matter, because she participated in many community activities related to church and philanthropies, and was even a kind of substitute mother for her younger sister, Ruth, and Ruth's four children.
>
> One day, when Ruth came home, she found Mary lying on the couch. "Guess what?" Mary said. "The doctor found a lump in my breast. I'm going into the hospital." While Mary seemed very casual the lesion turned out to be anything but benign. The diagnosis was inflammatory carcinoma, with mid-spine bony metastasis in addition to lymph node involvement. This meant anatomical Stage 3, despite absence of clinical symptoms. Rapid growth indicated that clinical Stage 2 was appropriate. An oophorectomy was performed.
>
> Mary readily talked about the diagnosis, but was not prepared to consider implications. This meant second-order denial. She had never been away from work very long over a 30-year span, and it was somewhat difficult to tolerate inactivity and restlessness. She had no pain. She coped by watching TV, talking with visitors, and going on short excursions with her nieces and nephews. Later, it was learned that she slept poorly, ate much less than before, and was privately very discouraged by lack of progress. Overtly, however, she expected to be out of work for about a month, then for a year, while she convalesced. This estimate about time perspective increased along with various symptoms. However, she had far milder symptoms than her anatomical staging and x-rays suggested. In fact, the cancer had spread to other bones at about the same time as Mary went back to work! To her, spread meant that the other breast might become involved. Since it showed no masses, dissemination was somewhat academic to her, except for the fact that other bones *were* implicated. So she returned to work.
>
> Radiation caused more fatigue, insomnia, and shortness of breath. Nevertheless, she kept up work, even at the price of having more pain (psychosocial Stage 2). But her courageous program gradually failed. She no longer talked about full recovery. "If I make any progress, I expect that it will be very slow." It was an understatement. The family was immensely supportive.

Pain now became an obtrusive problem. Mary was finally forced to give up work and move in with Ruth and her family (psychosocial Stage 3). Just about everything became an effort. More medication was necessary. However, although she had nowhere to go, Mary insisted upon getting out of bed each morning at the time she usually got ready for work. She hesitated asking physicians about anything, saying that they must be too busy. The fact was that she wanted to know nothing, but how to get back to her nonexistent job. At times, however, she remarked, "I know I'm supposed to be getting better, but I know I'm not."

Decline and deterioration were unmistakable, although she still made occasional trips outside the house. However, she became uncharacteristically irritable, possibly related to lack of sleep. She brushed aside questions about her health, saying that it was all up to her doctors. There was nothing she could do about it.

Within a few weeks, preterminality could no longer be avoided. Irritability gave way to a kind of tranquillity, in which she did not seem to resent her lack of job and independence. On one occasion, when her sister hesitated about going out, Mary said, "Please go. I know that I'm going to die. There's really nothing more for you to do." This was a statement of fact, not one of despair. When visitors came, as many did, she groomed herself well, took medication beforehand, and gave the appearance of still being relatively healthy. But she knew better, as did the family. One night, just as morning was beginning to dawn, she asked Ruth for some warm milk and medication to help her sleep. Then she turned out the lights, and never awakened. After her death, it was found that she had planned specifically for disposition of money and property, asking only that there be no dispute about her possessions. This wish was honored.

IMPORTANCE OF PSYCHOSOCIAL STAGING

The purpose of adding psychosocial staging to the already byzantine logic of anatomical and clinical staging is to provide a comprehensive context for any patient who has or has had cancer. It is essential for judging how seriously morale has been affected, since morale is easier to maintain when physical and psychosocial factors are kept under control. Psychosocial staging does not encourage the myth that tumors grow independently or in isolation. No one can be insulated, except by strategic avoidance or, in the case of physicians, monocular preoccupation with laboratory findings. If resources can be mobilized to preserve mitigation and accommodation (psychosocial Stage 2) as long as possible, then a cancer patient can be kept alive as a person even longer than justified by anatomical diagnosis. Unfortunately, some cancer patients are tacitly given up, or even pushed into psychosocial Stage 3 long before they are ready. When this happens, it is likely to be a sign of premature anticipatory grief.

Anatomical and clinical staging depend on tests and symptoms. Psychosocial staging depends only on listening or observing. For example, when a physician says, "Nothing else can be done at this time," he supposedly means that there is a need for further treatment, but that his therapeutic cupboard is bare. The patient is automatically consigned to decline and deterioration, regardless of how that patient may feel. Remarks, such as, "I don't think she can be taken care of at home," are even more pessimistic, but just as typical of a specific psychosocial stage, in this case, psychosocial Stage 4. Physicians are also active members of a patient's psychosocial context, whether they like it or not. Their attitudes reflect a coping style, as well as the psychosocial stage that they believe the patient is in.

Psychosocial staging puts flesh on the bare bones of clinicoanatomical staging. It is already implicit in what physicians now do, just as clinical staging is based on considerations other than those observable under the microscope. Palliative care should not be confined to the medical mummery that usually accompanies preterminality and terminality. Pain relief itself works better when combined with other activities.

The psychological autopsy is an exercise that recalls and reconstructs circumstances surrounding the preterminal and terminal stage, helping to recognize ways in which a patient's social identity might have been better preserved.[21] Now, if the psychological autopsy makes sense, then it is doubly advisable to use psychosocial staging and social assessment for any patient at any anatomical or clinical stage whom we want to keep alive as a responsible being, far beyond the closed loops and whorls of anatomy and clinical boundaries.

REFERENCES

1 Schulz, M., "Clinical Staging of Cancer and End Result Reporting," in *Cancer—A Manual for Practitioners,* 4th ed., American Cancer Society, Boston, 1968, chap. 7, pp. 53–66.

2 Terry, R., "Pathology of Cancer," in *Clinical Oncology for Medical Students and Physicians: A Multi-disciplinary Approach,* American Cancer Society, 4th ed., Rochester, N.Y., 1974, chap. II, pp. 26–47.

3 James, A., *Cancer Prognosis Manual,* American Cancer Society Publication, 2d ed., Boston, 1966.

4 Feinstein, A. R., "A New Staging System for Cancer and Reappraisal of 'Early' Treatment and 'Cure' by Radical Surgery," *New England Journal of Medicine,* **249**: 747–753, Oct. 3, 1968.

5a Feinstein, A., *Clinical Judgment,* The Williams and Wilkins Company, Baltimore, 1967.

5b Feinstein, A. R., J. A. Pritchett, and C. R. Schimpff, "The Epidemiology of Cancer Therapy, II. The Clinical Course: Data, Decisions and Temporal Demarcations," *Archives of Internal Medicine,* **123**: 323–344, March 1969.

6 Weisman, A., and J. W. Worden, "Psychosocial Analysis of Cancer Deaths," *Omega* **6**(1): 61–75, 1975.

7 Kastenbaum, R., and B. Kastenbaum, "Hope, Survival, and the Caring Environment," in *Prediction of Life Span,* E. Palmore and F. Jeffers (eds.), Heath Lexington Books, Lexington, Mass., 1971, chap. 19, pp. 249–271.

8   Weisman, A., and J. W. Worden, "Existential Plight of Cancer Patients," *International Journal of Psychiatry in Medicine,* 7(1): 1–15, 1976–1977.

9   Krant, M., *Dying and Dignity,* Charles C Thomas, Springfield, Ill., 1974.

10 Schonfield, J., "Psychological Factors Related to Delayed Return to an Earlier Life-Style in Successfully Treated Cancer Patients," *Journal of Psychosomatic Research,* 16: 41–46, 1972.

11 Schottenfeld, D., and G. Robbins, "Quality of Survival among Patients Who Have Had Radical Mastectomy," *Cancer,* 26: 650–654, 1970.

12 Cope, O., *The Breast: Its Problems, enign and Malignant,* Houghton, Mifflin Company, Boston, 1977.

13 Weisman, A., and J. W. Worden, "The Fallacy in Postmastectomy Depression," *American Journal of Medical Sciences,* 273 (2), 169–175, 1977.

14 Mount, B., "Problem of Caring for the Dying in a General Hospital: The Palliative Care Unit as a Possible Solution," *Canadian Medical Association Journal,* 115: 119–121, July 17, 1976.

15 Glaser, B. G., and A. L. Strauss, *Awareness of Dying,* Aldine Publishing Company, Chicago, 1965.

16 Hinton, J., "Bearing Cancer," *British Journal of Medical Psychology,* 46: 2, 105–113, 1973.

17 Costa, G., "Cachexia and the Systemic Effects of Tumors," in J. Holland and E. Frei (eds.), *Cancer Medicine,* Lea & Febiger, Philadelphia, 1973, chap. XVI-4, 1035–1043.

18 Kübler-Ross, E., *On Death and Dying,* The Macmillan Company, New York, 1969.

19 Urca, G., et al., "Morphine and Enkephalin: Analgesic and Epileptic Properties," *Science,* 197: (4298), 83–86, July 1, 1977.

20 Jaffe, L., and A. Jaffe, "Terminal Candor and the Coda Syndrome: A Tandem View of Fatal Illness," in H. Feifel (ed.), *New Meanings of Death,* McGraw-Hill Book Company, New York, 1977, chap. 11, pp. 195–211.

21 Weisman, A. D., *The Realization of Death: A Guide for the Psychological Autopsy,* Jason Aronson, Inc., New York, 1974.

Chapter 8

Coping and Anticipatory Grief

Death symbolizes almost everything we are taught to deplore and fear in life. It is the antithesis of whatever we are supposed to struggle for. Unless one truly believes that this world is but an unruly anteroom leading to a more serene reincarnation, death and the obligation to die represent sickness, suffering, infirmity, retribution, devaluation, defeat, or decay.[1] It is at once disavowed and yet always before us. At the very least, death is a transition from somethingness to nothingness, beyond choice or control. At its worst, death cancels out everything good and epitomizes unavoidable evil. Little wonder, then, that in every culture humanity knows about, death is preceded and followed by sadness, bereavement, and complicated rituals befitting a mysterious, yet common calamity.[2]

Die we must, whether of disease, injury, decrepitude, or suicide. The only unanswered questions are *when* and *how.* Nevertheless, for such a natural and universal event, people also have a passion about immortality. Quite apart from belief in an afterlife, almost any healthy or not-so-healthy human being insists upon a "not yet" for personal death, while accepting the inexorable fact of death as a biological necessity.[3]

My theme in this chapter is that form of coping with imminent death called "anticipatory grief." Its function is to rehearse the bereavement process. To anticipate a grief is to cope in advance with an inevitable loss, an event that commonly arises with preterminal and terminal cancer. This stage of cancer is a grave plight, not just for the patient, but for survivors-to-be. It is strange that we have no widely accepted, commonly used term for people who are soon to be widows, widowers, or orphans, even though it is a lonely death, indeed, that arouses no grief in anyone. Surely, before-death survivors have a set of attributes and roles, just as they have after death, when someone closely related dies. But the complicated rituals and taboos that follow death are less evident before death, possibly because inevitability is so difficult to accept, until it happens.

If fear of death comes from every other fear that humanity faces, then *anticipatory grief is fear of bereavement.* The prospect of "coming to grief" or being bereft is an unbearable threat. Consequently, it is pushed aside, rationalized, split into smaller parts, or dealt with by still other forms of Cope.

ANTICIPATORY GRIEF AND A BETTER BEREAVEMENT

I shall not discuss the long-term consequences of bereavement.[4] There are many publications about mourning and grief, some based on what to do and when to do it, although clinical and statistical studies are also available.[5,6] Bereavement, it seems, is an inviting field.

Practically every article about bereavement offers an outline of different stages and diagnostic events that people are supposed to pass through until resolution is reached.[7] However, other than grief itself, I find it difficult to recognize any uniformly specific stages or types of symptoms, which are timed to certain periods after death. This should not be surprising, considering how unique relationships can be, and how diverse feelings are. Behavior can be labeled, of course, but prescribed activities befitting a mourner are usually decided by custom, not always by how that person actually feels.

Coping with cancer cannot ignore the possibility that treatment will be unsuccessful. Coping with this outcome means that forewarning and anticipatory grief is frequent enough to merit more attention than it has received.[8] Like coping itself, no antemortem behavior is universal, and like bereavement itself, no regularity can be predicted. Manifest and occult signs of bereavement vary. As a rule, however, anticipatory grief cannot and does not exempt survivors from all sadness in advance. But it does provide a means of setting in motion a unique process of relinquishing a key person, and then filling a void. Not everyone dies hard, as Buckley and Michaels point out.[9] Some families draw together, mustering strengths, and joining strategies. Others fall apart, with each member going a separate way. Usually, anticipatory grief starts with the diagnosis, but does not really come into focus until psychosocial stages 3 and 4, because it is easier to mitigate earlier.

It is presumptuous to describe the "normal" process of bereavement, and to tell families and significant others how they should respond during anticipatory grief. For some, the only Cope is uncontrolled weeping and mourning, as if the patient (and their kin or spouse) were already dead. Coping, in this situation, is catharsis. At the other extreme, coping is shown by hypercontrol and matter-of-factness that correspond more to cultural norms and personality traits than to depth of feeling. Grief can be measured only by what goes on inside. Anticipatory grief is very private. Local custom, cultural sanctions, and even ethnic expectations do help direct the onset and duration of bereavement.[10]

How long is normal grief? Duration in specific time periods is an artifact. It is like asking how high is up. "Up" is only a direction which might be followed. Manifest signs of bereavement disappear in a matter of months; most people are back at their usual way of life much earlier. But occult bereavement can continue throughout the remainder of life, even though survivors sometimes can scarcely recall more than a fleeting, fragmentary image of the person who died.

Hospital professionals, especially medical staff, tend to regard survivors-to-be as people who merely escort patients, and sometimes tarry long enough to ask a few apologetic questions. They seemingly serve no special function, either in coping with cancer, or in having frailties that require intervention, information, or solace. That some of this attitude is now changing is another sign of an alert consumerism, along with self-help and demystification of medicine and its practitioners. Representing this change are families of preterminal patients who now form groups in various hospitals and communities in order to share experiences, advise, and console. There are clubs for widows and for couples who have lost a child to cancer. Laudable as this is, however, much more is required to serve the needs found in anticipatory grief. Preparation or at least having an opportunity to exchange and express ideas and feelings may ameliorate some of the painful loss that will follow.

In one of the few extant studies of anticipatory grief, Glick, Weiss, and Parkes found that forewarning of a husband's death helped some widows recover and find new resources earlier than if the death occurred suddenly.[11] While these women were just as shocked at the time of death, denial occurred much less often than in women whose husbands died unexpectedly. Untimely deaths may be hard to take, because what, after all, is a "timely" death? Such deaths, however, are not always calamitous.[12] As with other kinds of pain, forewarning of death lessens duration and intensity of grief, while not, of course, eliminating it entirely or providing a mourning without tears. Death still seems abrupt and shocking, even though survivors-to-be are wholly aware of the prognosis.

In my opinion, preterminal patients are often better prepared to deal with their own demise than are members of their family. Consequently, part of the coping process which fosters a better death consists of enlisting cooperation of the *patient* to support the spouse during the difficult periods. It also helps the patient maintain a somewhat steady social role, resembling that regularly filled in the past.

Engel, Schmale, and others postulated a "giving up/given up" syndrome many years ago, in connection with hospitalized patients.[13] Schmale pursued this connection further in his work with cancer patients, showing how, in some cases, somatic illness follows a psychological stress, especially a loss or death.[14] I believe that there is still insufficient information to forge a firm link between "giving up/given up" and cancer, just as I do about other etiological hypotheses. Nevertheless, various illnesses are reported to be more frequent among survivors than in matched comparison groups.[15] The inference seems clear: Better anticipatory resolution might not only reduce prolonged bereavement, but eliminate secondary physical and psychological aberrance later on.

Bereavement is erroneously regarded as a thoroughly natural phenomenon, hardly a process, that usually disappears after a time without special attention. This may be because very few survivors seek psychiatric aid or counseling until many months, if not years, have elapsed. Abnormal grief and delayed mourning are, however, well-recognized manifestations of problems in relinquishing a significant other.[16] But attenuating grief through anticipatory coping is still a new idea. It is *not* synonymous with mere forewarning, pessimism, or a long vigil at the bedside.

Most people do not realize that mourning can be muted and be no less sincere, respectful, or symbolic of deep love. Disruption, of course, is still disruption. But plans can be made, distress confronted, problems considered, coping strategies contemplated, so that forewarning through anticipatory grief becomes a useful period. Mourning will occur; shock is still there, even among the best prepared potential survivors. But it is manageable. One man, for example, said that the full impact of his wife's death first struck him when the funeral home aide came to take her body away. Because her death was expected, they shared much in anticipation of the inexorable. She taught him many things about the household and their finances that she had always taken care of. After the impact of actual death, he was somewhat disabled by her absence, very lonely, but much less devastated than might have been expected, considering his dependence. He mourned deeply, observed customs, and gradually resumed a different kind of life, while retaining precious memories. I do not know whether forewarning itself always shortens bereavement, because many other coping factors come together through traditional observances and in mourning proper.

Past regrets, pessimism, and marital problems prior to cancer do make a significant difference in coping effectiveness. It is often difficult to tell how a couple actually got along through the years, when one spouse is very ill and needs the help of the other. That a couple stayed married is just a statistic. One woman, dying of cancer, always praised her dutiful, loyal husband who visited every day. He seemed completely devoted, except for certain equivocal signs of being breezier than most husbands are in a similar plight, which observers noted to themselves. After her death, a sister reported acidly that the husband had been having an affair with a much younger woman. She suspected that her sister knew, but nothing was ever brought into the open. Thus, his attentiveness was suspect. I assume there was little anticipatory grief, although she was touched by his apparent concern and love.

Classic psychoanalytic theory would have us believe that ambivalence toward the deceased is a most decisive factor in postmortem melancholia, as opposed to reactive depression.[17] I doubt this hypothesis, because there are so few deep relationships without ambivalence. Moreover, depressions of all kinds occur with and without specific connection with the death of a significant other.[18] Anniversary reactions are intriguing.[19] However, I suspect not only that many important anniversaries go unnoticed, but that some so-called anniversary reactions to an earlier loss or death are forced and artificial.

Nevertheless, to love is to fear losing the person loved. Grief and love are mirror images. Even the threat of separation stirs up sadness, anger, hopelessness, and anxiety. It may at times rekindle love, as might have happened with the husband who was having an affair. Self-reliant people will probably continue to cope effectively, while the very dependent spouse has more to lose, and therefore copes less well. Contrary to psychoanalytic theory, then, actual loss is apt to be more painful when the survivor is highly dependent, and hardly ambivalent at all. If true, then bereavement can start earlier, and perhaps through effective anticipation, lead to a better death, even an appropriate death. If this happens, a better bereavement, with fewer complications for survivors, might be expected. The help of the soon-to-be-deceased is a resource seldom used.

APPROPRIATE DEATH

Better bereavement should be the consequence of a better death. In effect, this means better anticipatory coping, less distress, fewer unresolved problems, more support, and fuller preparation. These preliminary procedures take the edge off dismay and horror out of actual loss, and subsequently lead to milder mourning and bereavement.

Most people would postpone death and its realization as long as possible. This reasonable attitude is different from maintaining that death can *never* be acceptable or appropriate, except for those who deserve it or seek quiet release from suffering and travail. Contrary to entrenched beliefs, some deaths are or could be made more acceptable to all concerned, but especially the primary patient. Furthermore, there are even qualities and conditions that could enhance or endow good deaths with a conviction of appropriateness.[20] Conceivably, and practically, when death is inevitable, it is still possible to improve the quality of life in such a way that dying proceeds at its own pace, without hastening its course, transforming death into a befitting, beneficent act.

An appropriate death has these four characteristics: *awareness, acceptability, propriety,* and *timeliness.* It need not be particularly propitious, ideal, or romantic. And it happens to regular people, not to fictional characters. Very simply, an appropriate death begins when a dying patient comes to realize that nothing more can or should be done. The decision may be belated, but the groundwork is laid much earlier, when decline and deterioration are first recognized. Everything that might have bedevilled, compromised, or needlessly prolonged existence has already been dealt with. Persistent problems are resolved or left comfortably in limbo. It is time to die.

The principal prerequisites for an appropriate death are:

1 Care: This consists of adequate symptom relief, comfort, and support by and of significant others.

2 Control: The patient collaborates, even if it is simply to yield control over decisions during the preterminal stage.

3 Composure: It is time to be calm and collected. Emotional extremes are reduced, but not so totally obliviated that a patient cannot respond. Mildness is the key quality, but nevertheless, there is ample room for sympathy, impatience, resentment, and so forth. Sometimes, a patient prefers to be kept stuporous. If so, this, too, is a choice, but should not be confused with composure.

4 Communication: A well-informed patient generally does better because the essence of mutuality is communication. Needs are made known, and when it is not possible to satisfy those needs, reasons can be made clear, compassionate, and compromises reached.

5 Continuity: A patient can be kept alive as a person by preserving token functions of normal life. In doing so, the transition from one psychosocial stage to another is smoother.

6 Closure: Residual problems are resolved or redefined. Some patients are ready to die before their body lets them go. Others are implacable to the end, depending on the Cope used earlier. Nevertheless, although it is time to die, time is no longer important.

An appropriate death presumes good care and management by others. The element of mutuality is continuous, permitting gradual surrender while actively relinquishing hold. The demise becomes a necessary but acceptable consequence. Conventional measurement of time by clock or calendar drops away. An hour seems like a few minutes or several days. Hastening the dying process, therefore, is only a forensic problem for professionals, and an emotional problem for survivors-to-be, who must stand by, grief-stricken and quivering with indecision.[21]

Assuming that pain relief is good, and that a patient has not been devaluated during treatment, time is as meaningless as the future. The best deaths are those that a person might have accepted and chosen, had there been a choice.[22] A good death and better bereavement begin with better coping, especially by maintaining high morale (see Chapter 10) and encouraging firm support of and by significant others.

HOW TO REACH AN APPROPRIATE DEATH

An appropriate death is one we can live with. It is part of the process of being alive. It is good coping extended as far as possible. Characteristics of awareness, acceptability, propriety, and timeliness, however, need specific "instructions" or directions, in addition to prerequisites. I recognize that the following precepts for patients are easier to state than to fulfill:

1 Avoid avoidances. Denial is effective only to a limited degree.
2 Confront what must be confronted, and correct whatever is realistic and practical.
3 Resolve remaining conflicts and concerns, or at least be sure what they are.
4 Trust your own sense of reality, using your own resources as far as possible.
5 Learn to trust others when they deserve it.
6 Seek out and use competent help when necessary or when offered.
7 Insist upon decent medical management on your own terms.
8 Communicate openly, as never before, especially with significant others.
9 Remember that this period now facing you should be the justification for having lived in the first place. Your death belongs to you, and must be symbolic of you at the highest level attainable.
10 Others die, too, with your death. Permit them to grieve.

As I implied in Chapter 1, *hope is the precondition of good coping, but morale is its outcome.* Because people are less than paragons, there is often a mixture of high morale, which fuses self-esteem, solidarity of values, and belief in what one is trying to be and do, with such signs of demoralization as apathy, exhaustion, futility, frustration, and resentment.

GOOD CANDIDATES FOR A BAD DEATH

How do we recognize cancer patients in whom the quantum of vulnerability almost ensures a bad death? That incurability is not the issue is shown by a recent study of 32 men, all of whom died of lung cancer. Each patient was seen within 10 days of the initial diagnosis, then followed regularly for at least 6 months, and periodically thereafter.

I must interpolate how difficult it is to carry out significant and satisfactory follow-up evaluations, with frequent interviews of sufficient numbers of patients and families. With rare exceptions, one depends on secondary sources, such as family and friends, for later information after initial contact, or else first meets a patient during the preterminal and terminal stages. Consequently, private attitudes and perceptions are apt to be swayed by circumstances, retrospective wish fulfillment, or a disposition to conform with community expectations. Long after death, a survivor may revise an earlier opinion, and inaccurately recall events. An investigator must be circumspect as well as skeptical.

Most of these men died outside of the Massachusetts General Hospital. This is not unusual. New cancer patients are often seen in a large medical center, but terminal care is the function of local physicians, community hospitals, nursing homes, and family members. Research associates, all social workers, had kept in touch and offered prompt condolences to the widows. Several months later, they made a home visit to evaluate bereavement of the widow, and to learn more about the former patient's final weeks and days.

The psychosocial criteria used to determine a good, bad, or equivocal death were the following:

Medication needed
Relief of symptoms
Doctor-patient relationship
Attitude toward death, if known
Preterminal expressions of distress
Communication with significant others
Autonomy and control
Support needed and available
Denial and avoidance of critical issues

Eleven men fulfilled criteria for a good death, eleven others for a bad death, and ten remaining were considered to have equivocal deaths, that is, neither good nor bad according to their scores.

More subtle nuances of feeling, attitudes, or relationships could not be judged with confidence, for reasons already given. While it was not possible to do more than conjecture about appropriate death, there was evidence for judging whether a good, bad, or equivocal death had occurred. These deaths allowed us to see how candidates for a *bad* death might be recognized earlier:

Lower socioeconomic status
Uncertain about an afterlife

More pessimistic
More past regrets
Alienation from others
Cope by withdrawal (12), suppression (4), and blame (13)
Dejection and resentment
More denial at all times
Needed more medication
Little sense of autonomy or control
Talked hardly at all
Did not die at place of choice

Note that age and physical symptoms did not appear to differentiate good and bad deaths. Pain medication was amply available for all, but the bad death patients still seemed to need more. Whether their need was actually for pain relief remains uncertain. There were other factors, such as doctor-patient relationship and attitude toward death, which might also have affected the patient's overall response. Direct daily personal contact would have been necessary, were these highly subjective data to be defined and measured accurately.

From the physical standpoint, good and bad deaths were found in an equal number of patients with oat cell carcinoma, a particularly resistant and rapidly growing malignancy. This indicates that the histology or anatomical lesion is not the only critical factor. However, good death patients had more squamous cell cancers which had been diagnosed at an earlier anatomical stage. Since squamous cell patients usually live longer, this finding suggests that afflicted patients might have had more time to accommodate before deteriorating. Nevertheless, older men were just as reluctant as younger men about dying. Conversely, it might be said that younger to middle-aged men could accept death as freely as older men.

The total survival period for all patients ranged from about one month to over a year. Unfortunate physical complications did influence the length and quality of life in some cases. For example, one fairly young man who had a very supportive family, devoted wife, and skilled physician developed perforation of a bronchus shortly after starting radiation therapy. He had incredible distress before succumbing in a very short time. Had he been able to withstand this complication, it was wholly possible, given his psychosocial assets, that he might have had a good death, instead of the suffering he was forced to endure.

Psychosocial factors do, of course, interlock. A man without skills who becomes sick and disabled undergoes diminished self-esteem as well as finances. In contrast, a business or professional man with private means and a personal physician can at least make needs known, with confidence that his wishes will be heeded, including death at the place of choice.

We have little absolute information about the effect of psychosocial factors on longevity, but the question *could* be investigated, were cancerologists inclined to seek and record such information.[23] It is certain that psychosocial factors change the quality, if not the duration, of life. Feasibly, by suitable interventions, better ways of coping might shift equivocal deaths into better deaths, and edge bad deaths into equivocal deaths.

Few patients or families ask the impossible. For example, no widow in this study blamed the physician because her husband died. Physicians were faulted for allegedly callous, indifferent, overly optimistic, or inconsiderate behavior, which could easily have been rectified. Good-death families even recalled small favors, which had a lasting effect beyond the time and effort needed. In bad-death families, doctors were reported to be unavailable, too busy, and even too sanguine. They often gave palliative treatment which inflicted more suffering than benefit.

Some things are beyond help, and cannot be changed by any known means. But matters such as adequate information, availability, and enduring support are quite modest and very inexpensive. Little is asked, and whatever is given goes a long way. Appropriate death is not just for a very few. A better death for patients who cope effectively, and use resources well, is attainable by practically everyone who is willing to participate, and accept efforts of others.

PRUDERY AND DEATH

Death is, admittedly, best considered from a distance, whether with a sense of horror or fascination. Many of those who find death a fashionable topic would be repelled by the sights, smells, sounds, and symptoms of patients sick and on the threshold of extinction. Those who are concerned with coping and cancer would prefer the more positive attitude, which consists of hope, morale, optimism, and, to be sure, absolute cure. I am one of them. But I also know that until one can become aware, accept, and fulfill some of the criteria and instructions for an appropriate death, even in running everyday life, then satisfactory coping with cancer is somewhat illusory. Denial, pretense, and pseudooptimism do not promote the positive side of cancer care, which requires candor and compassion. The same attitude should apply to bereavement, which is a deep fear of losing and being lost to someone significant whom we love.

There is a prudery about death that resembles sexual prudery. That sex and death evoke major taboos is by now a trite observation. Both appeal to the negative side of society's favorite topics. There is a ringing validity in Gorer's trenchant phrase, "pornography of death."[24] Sexual pornography can be shown to have parallels in death pornography. We are urged to suppress the bleak fact of death, just as sexuality is disguised in various ways. Furthermore, people often have a more prudish attitude toward death as a personal reality than they do about flagrant sexual display. Death is romanticized, spoken about in pious platitudes, or laughed aside with gallows humor. Otherwise, it evokes a shudder. That it is not always so forbidding is shown by the differences between good deaths and bad deaths.

The pornography of sex and death share other common traits which combine and resolve intolerable conflicts between the forbidden and the fascinating. For example, because sexual conflicts are almost universal, pornography shows a world in which these problems are not confronted, but rather one in which substitute fantasies replace conflicts and are exploited. Death pornography also joins the dreadful and the desirable, but it too exploits a fantasy that death is not inexorable. The graveyard waits for everyone, but not yet.

Scatology and eschatology have more in common than their sound. Although prudery insists otherwise, obscenity is not the same as pornography. If one can separate the two in our thoughts, then pornography is only a make-believe world in which women are insatiable, men are inexhaustible, desire is perpetual, and death is impossible. A world without death, such as prudery would support, is pornographic, not miraculous. When stripped of dignity, wholesome awareness, morale, propriety, or timeliness, death can be very obscene, as, indeed, it is in warfare, torture, holocausts, and so forth. There is no love in sexual pornography, and probably none in death pornography. Neither is there failure, frustration, vulnerability, or bereavement. No coping is required because death is excluded.

Coping and bereavement belong to the burden of being alive in a real world, not one in which essential elements are suppressed, disguised, diluted, or rendered pornographic. Anticipatory grief foreshadows the task of coping with having loved. To foreswear such grief is an act of prudery that avoids an ultimate fact or concern. To accept death as our personal obligation cuts through pretense, eliminates make-believe fantasies, and helps cope better with adversity.

REFERENCES

1   Feifel, H. (ed.), *The Meaning of Death,* McGraw-Hill Book Company, New York, 1959.

2   Blauner, R., "Death and Social Structure," *Psychiatry,* **29:** 378–394, November 1966.

3   Parkes, C., *Bereavement: Studies of Grief in Adult Life,* International Universities Press, Inc., New York, 1972.

4   Jackson, E. N., *Understanding Grief,* Abingdon Press, New York, 1957.

5   Clayton, P., L. Desmarais, and G. Winokur, "A Study of Normal Bereavement," *American Journal of Psychiatry,* **125:** 64–74, August 1968.

6   Westberg, G., *Minister and Doctor Meet,* Harper & Row Publishers, Incorporated, New York, 1961.

7   Schoenberg, B., A. Carr, A. Kutscher, D. Peretz, and I. Goldberg, (eds.), *Anticipatory Grief,* Columbia University Press, New York and London, 1974.

8   Weisman, A., "Is Mourning Necessary?" in B. Schoenberg, A. Carr, A. Kutscher, D. Peretz, and I. Goldberg (eds.), *Anticipatory Grief,* Columbia University Press, New York, 1974, pp. 14–18.

9   Buckley, I., and R. Michaels, "Variations on a Theme: Case Reports from Cancer Care," in Schoenberg, B., A. Carr, A. Kutscher, D. Peretz, and I. Goldberg, (eds.), *Anticipatory Grief,* Columbia University Press, New York and London, 1974, pp. 135–153.

10 Pine, V., et al. (eds.), *Acute Grief and the Funeral,* Charles C Thomas, Springfield, Ill., 1976.

11 Glick, I., R. Weiss, and C. Parkes, *The First Year of Bereavement,* John Wiley & Sons, New York, 1974.

12 Weisman, A., "Coping with Untimely Death," *Psychiatry,* **36:** 366–377, November 1973.

13 Engel, G., and A. Schmale, "Psychoanalytic Theory of Somatic Disorder," *Journal of American Psychoanalytic Association,* **15:** 344–365, 1967.

14 Schmale, A., "Relationship of Separation and Depression to Disease," *Psychosomatic Medicine,* **XX:** 4, 259–277, 1958.

15 Dewi Rees, W., "Bereavement and Illness," in Schoenberg, B., A. Carr, D. Peretz, and A. Kutscher, (eds.), *Psychosocial Aspects of Terminal Care,* Columbia University Press, New York and London, 1972, pp. 210–220.

16 Volkan, V., "Typical Findings in Pathological Grief," *Psychiatric Quarterly,* **44:** 231–250, 1970.

17 Freud, S., *Mourning and Melancholia,* Standard Edition, Vol. XIV, Hogarth Press, London, 1957, pp. 237–258.

18 Leff, M., J. Roatch, and W. Bunney, "Environmental Factors Preceding the Onset of Severe Depressions," *Psychiatry,* **33**(3): 293–311, 1970.

19 Hilgard, J., "Depressive and Psychotic States as Anniversaries to Sibling Death in Childhood," in E. Shneidman & M. Ortega (eds.), *Aspects of Depression,* Little, Brown and Company, Boston, 1969, pp. 197–211.

20 "The Question of Appropriate Death," in Weisman, A., *The Realization of Death,* Jason Aronson, New York and London, 1974, pp. 138–152.

21 Veatch, R., *Death, Dying and Biological Revolution: Our Last Quest for Responsibility,* Yale University Press, New Haven and London, 1976.

22 Weisman, A., "The Dying Patient," in R. Pasnau (ed.), *Consultation—Liaison Psychiatry,* Grune & Stratton, Inc., New York, 1975, pp. 237–244.

23 Palmore, E., and F. Jeffers. (eds.), *Prediction of Life Span,* Heath Lexington Books, Lexington, Mass., 1971.

24 Gorer, Geoffrey, "The Pornography of Death," in W. Phillips and P. Rahv (eds.), *Modern Writing,* New York: McGraw-Hill, 1959, pp. 157–188.

Coping and Countercoping

Is competent and comprehensive cancer care restricted to cutting, burning, or poisoning tissues? Obviously not, yet to many people, not excluding physicians, the function of a psychiatrist is defined in just about the same scurrilous way. "I don't want my patient to get upset" implies that merely talking with a cancer patient will, in itself, create enormous turmoil. "What can psychiatrists do anyway?" is a common, but rhetorical question to which few who ask will stop to hear an answer. As shown in Chapter 8, one of the principal complaints of cancer survivors, and presumably of patients who underwent a bad death, is that the attending physician was too busy, preoccupied, optimistic, or remote to care much about anything beyond the cancer or prescription of drugs. The cancer is a lesion disembodied from the sick person and the family. That psychosocial problems might contribute to overall distress, or that informed counseling might clarify or even help at any stage, is seldom considered. Even the idea that cancer patients must cope with a variety of problems beyond the cancer is an alien notion for many physicians.

ARE PSYCHIATRISTS NECESSARY?

Like most yes or no questions, the answer must be qualified. Most large hospitals have psychiatric services. Unfortunately, it is often true that psychiatrists are uninterested and, therefore, lack experience with cancer patients. It is also true that other hospital professionals, such as social workers, chaplains, and nurse clinicians know more, care more, and already have a more established and acceptable role in providing psychosocial assistance.

What then might a psychiatrist really do, as one of a cluster of professionals looking after distressed cancer patients? For an answer, we already have the encouraging example of liaison psychiatry in general hospitals.[1] Liaison psychiatry is primarily concerned with how physical illness impinges on the human condition, or, conversely, how a patient's psychosocial plight puts pressure on physical well-being. It is a prototype for cancer care. Liaison psychiatrists participate in the management of problem patients on the basis of formulation as well as insight.

Hackett urges psychiatrists to get off the shores and swim in the mainstream of medicine.[2] I heartily agree, especially when psychiatrists are profligate with pronouncements and conclusions, based only on speculation about a very few, possibly exceptional cancer patients. But cancer specialists for their part, too, have not been eager to recognize or develop psychosocial skills, nor have they fully accepted the contribution of coping better with manifold distress.

Communication between cancerologists and liaison psychiatrists, other than on a personal basis of friendship, is intermittent at best. Collaboration in the care of patients is very rare. Cancer registries never report psychosocial data, and information about survival is largely statistical. Only a few investigators seem to consider quality of life, social adjustment, ability to work, or return to a reasonable status after treatment. Screening for psychosocial risk is embryonic. Moreover, cancer patients will stoically accept painful procedures of dubious relevance and yet may resist and rebuff almost any physician who announces that he or she is also a psychiatrist. "Why are you seeing me? Does my doctor think I'm imagining all this? Am I losing my mind, is that it? No, Doctor, I agree that for some people, psychiatry might help, but you shouldn't waste your time here, when others need you." As a rule, cancer patients who are most distressed are often those who are most resistant, while patients with lower distress levels are rather eager to converse and to confide in psychiatric consultants. A psychiatrist, concerned about how people cope or undergo distress related to cancer, is very often the unmentionable meeting the unmotivated.

A competent, conscientious psychiatrist or clinical psychologist does not create, aggravate, foment problems or unhinge the emotionally unstable. The psychiatrist may only discover or reveal psychosocial dimensions in cancer that routine workup fails to look for. If found, areas of concern or discord still may be considered irrelevant or trivial. Suppose, for example, a woman develops cancer of the ovary at the age when her mother died of the same disease. It is not a mere coincidence, but a special situation that may handicap the patient in her efforts to cope. Unlike the usual reason for calling a psychiatric consultant, psychosocial distress does not spring noisily into being and turn the patient into a "management problem."

Psychiatrists could never see more than a small fraction of cancer patients anyway. Their major role, beyond that of liaison, is to find psychological "pressure points" that bear further investigation. Beyond this, however, a cancer psychiatrist's vocation would at best formulate and set into motion an individualized program that is intended to fortify or correct existing coping strategies. I call such interventions "countercoping."

INTERVENTION AND COUNTERCOPING

The psychiatrist has no axe to grind or need to apologize for a style of thinking. The main purpose of psychosocial intervention is to help vulnerable cancer patients accommodate better, mitigate more effectively, and fit into their prevailing plight with less distress. The principles of countercoping are abstracted from observations of what works best. Consequently, such principles are pragmatic, existential, and operational. Objectives are simple: to restore a sense of choice, improve morale, and ameliorate the consequences of being a cancer patient.

What a psychiatrist does, or, more accurately, what anyone with sufficient training and concern could do, is to find out how a cancer patient customarily copes with different kinds of problems. Then by using appropriate countercoping strategies, the patient is helped to alleviate, neutralize, reinterpret, or resolve problematic situations.

My caution about being lured into the outer space of psychodynamic cosmology is the result of having lived through the promise and disappointment of psychosomatic medicine following World War II. The apparent connection between emotion, stress, and diseases of unknown etiology inspired profiles and typologies supposedly representing specific disease-prone personalities.[3] Cancer did not escape such categorical treatment, regardless of how diversified the neoplastic process proved to be.[4] It is feasible, of course, that turmoil tips the delicate balance of cellular, hormonal, genetic, and immune mechanisms, interfering and producing cancerous change. But the gap is very wide, as Fox points out.[5] We have no Isaac Newton to establish formulas for action at a distance between psychosocial distress and histological aberrations. So I leave the question of intermediary processes for the day when a more specific link between conflict and cancer can be clarified. Feasibility, meanwhile, is not fact. What I advocate is merely more comprehensive programs, based on psychological understanding, which will expand boundaries of cancer care.

Countercoping Complements Coping It should not be mistaken for "contracoping," which, I presume, would mean going against coping strategies. Countercoping is like counterpoint in music, which blends melodies together into basic harmony. The patient copes; the therapist countercopes; together, they work out a better fit.

Countercoping strategies are essentially *outcomes,* not techniques (see Table 6). With the exceptions of blame, shame, or imprudent, reckless behavior, each mode of countercoping corresponds to one or more Cope, described in Chapter 3. They range from active confrontation, giving more information, telling someone what to do, rephrasing the problem, or refraining from something, to more passive submission, silence, or temporary avoidance.

Countercoping can be done almost anywhere, in the office, at the bedside, even in corridors. But it is the countercoper, the one who intervenes, who establishes "technique." For this, I would abolish preconceived notions, and instead look for a therapist who has genuine interest and a sensitive, but precise, approach to evaluation and empathy. In fact, the four general outcomes should be exemplified in the personality of the therapist, by his or her capacity to respond compassionately and to improvise when

Table 6   Countercoping Strategies

A Clarification and control
1 Confront with salient problem and take appropriate action
2 Get or give more information
3 Redefine or reduce problems to manageable concerns
4 Consider alternative solutions

B Collaboration
1 Mutuality/constructive sharing of concern
2 Submit problems to judgment of another
3 Prevent impulsive actions or ill-considered behavior
4 Be more directive and active in the alliance

C Directed relief
1 Elicit catharsis and unburdening
2 Temporary avoidance and suppression
3 Encourage diversions that worked in the past
4 Suggest new tactics that relieve

D Cooling off
1 Modulate emotional extremes
2 Build morale through increased self-esteem
3 Rationalize and distract
4 Realistic resignation/be in silence

---

necessary. Reaching for too much may be self-defeating.

INTERVIEWING

Begin where the patient is, or with what there is concern about. Even the unmotivated patient seldom lacks discussable topics. Naturally, if a patient is too sick or sedated to participate, coping is minimal, and so is counter-coping. Every encounter is a new experience, because the here-and-now is all there is, except for forces pushing a patient from the past toward forces drawing him or her into the future.

> What problems do you expect as a result of being sick, or having an illness like yours? [Do not hesitate to use the word "cancer" if the physician has already spoken with the patient.]

> Look ahead a few weeks. What do you anticipate, judging by the things that have been hardest to deal with during the last week or so?

Questions usually phrase themselves, but should be focused on the present predicament or medical plight. Keep the patient at the center, despite temptations to digress. The patient's perceptions, however skewed, may be more informative than actual dates and facts. For example, instead of asking when a patient's parents died, ask what it was like when they died, or what the patient remembers most about the parents.

Talking with patients involves a style that is more readily absorbed and generated than taught and prescribed, even though volumes have been written about interviewing for various purposes.[6,7,8] Interviewing is really a rather cold word for the transaction between two people, one of whom is a patient. It is not, however, synonymous with psychosocial intervention, nor are countercoping strategies limited to data from interviews.

Countercoping uses the interviewer (therapist, intervener, etc.) as an instrument. The encounter is expectant and spontaneous, but seldom what one expects or anticipates. Consequently, the interviewer is revealed as often as the patient interviewed. If there is a good match, countercoping takes place in the midst of interviewing. If not, interviewing is pointless. Nevertheless, a few precepts will help the process of give-and-take:

1 Ask only open-ended questions, namely, those that cannot be answered with yes or no.

2 Do not hesitate to ask for clarification, even if the meaning seems obvious. "For instance?" "I'm not clear . . ." "In what respect?" tend to stress the individual, evoking an emotional response, not necessarily more exact information.

3 Empathy is seldom a natural gift, but can be acquired. Try to imagine different ways of looking at the same situation, picturing various feelings toward the same set of facts. Imagine yourself as the patient's "double."

4 Being overly sympathetic distorts as much as being overly rational and objective.

5 Paraphrase to understand better, not to parrot without feeling.

6 Forbearance may be rewarding. Respect a patient's reticence, and do not hurry.

7 Rephrase potential distress more tactfully: "Not everyone has the courage to admit being anxious or afraid. What has it been like for you?"

8 Do not hide behind a screen of silence or anonymity.

9 Do not be afraid to persist gently, but when a distraught patient closes off, retrace the topic in another way.

10 Choose activity over passivity, if a choice is called for, but then allow the patient to follow you at his or her pace.

11 Guard against mere chat by trying to measure or rank what is most relevant, real, or uppermost. Example: 'Who is your *best* friend?", "What bothered you *most* about that?", "How do you feel *now* as compared with, say, last week?", "What about the times when you felt really *good?*"

12 Tentative suggestions may draw out a reluctant patient, even to disagree. "Perhaps I'm wrong, but you seem to want to be by yourself as much as possible."

13 Clarify often, interpret seldom, never conjecture.

Examples:
"You felt as if there was no one to turn to." (Clarification)

"You didn't let anyone know how worried you were because you were afraid to get things out in the open and hear what you didn't want to hear." (Interpretation)

"You want to hear only good things, especially that everything is all a mistake, and that nothing has happened at all." (Conjecture)

DEBRIEFING

Self-interrogation after a session is not only an excellent discipline, but another precept that deserves more discussion. As a participant, the intervener should silently ask, "What did I do, and why did I do it that way?" or "What else could I have said or done?" Self-examination helps hone skills as well as disclosing tendencies that interfere with an honest exchange. For example, a very supportive therapist may not confront or clarify enough, while an overly eager therapist may plunge ahead, without noting its effect on the patient. Cooling off may calm the sympathetic listener more than the patient. Mere "show of interest" is not a strategy which can be deliberately followed; it is presumed, because there is no real alternative. Although one cannot confront and close off at the same time, it is common practice to allow feelings to emerge, then to become more rationally disposed, and seek further information, tacitly dispelling excessive emotion. If encouraged, no patient is likely to become more distressed.

All these considerations can be detected through self-examination and debriefing soon after a session. Otherwise, spontaneity and flavor, including much of the substance, quickly melt away. Onerous as it is, prompt recording is desirable. If not possible, then the intervener might jot down a few key words and cues for later reference: This is what I heard, said, sensed, or acted upon.

Debriefing has advantages over note taking, which is distracting and impersonal, or taped interviews, which are somewhat inconvenient and at best contain only words, not feelings, gestures, or unspoken observations. Debriefing is a dictated, detailed, candid summary of the entire transaction, emphasizing what the intervener thought, said, implied, or did in response to the patient. Naturally, a patient's comments and behavior are also included. Later, the report can be scrutinized in order to identify the patient's Cope and the intervener's strategies of countercoping. Surprisingly, debriefing that captures personal feelings and sentiments, even vagrant thoughts, usually turns out to be much more complete and informative than so-called process interviews. The best interviews are not mere question and answer, but narratives.[9] Here is a sample segment of debriefing, somewhat censored and very condensed:

> The patient looks very sick, as if he lost a lot of weight. Must have been a pretty strong man, but he seems a little confused, bored maybe. At least I don't feel any contact. He is very concrete but vague at the same time. Abstract ideas or questions don't get across, especially if they have something to do with the future. Maybe he just doesn't want to be bothered, or talk at all. I was very restless, wanting to end the session, right then and there. So I probably read something into his behavior that started with me. I felt as if I couldn't get anywhere. Where do I want to get? He didn't seem much interested, and neither was I.
>
> I asked something, I forget what, about the children. But he gave me a number, as if I'd asked how many children he had! That is certainly abstract enough. He seemed beyond caring, or intoxicated, both, maybe. At least I thought he didn't care until he turned away and gazed out the window, way out, beyond somewhere, certainly out of the room. I also saw that his eyes glistened with tears.
>
> This kind of man doesn't cry openly. He isn't so tough. Why am I concerned about how tough he is or isn't? Am I afraid of him? I'm worried about making him angry. But he's not angry, just sick. I settled by saying that it's hard for a vigorous man to be sick and not know what the future holds. That took in everything. He didn't even nod, or seem to hear me. I then asked what it was like to let people do things for him that he was accustomed to doing for himself. Sounds familiar.
>
> He denies feeling weak. But he is very weak, needs help just to get up

from a chair. He comes out with more denial: I just need time to recuperate from the operation. It is at least a reference to the future. Shows limited time perspective, but also redefines the present plight as a temporary interlude. Then he surprises me by saying that he bought a new car last week. He was in the hospital then. How come? It was really the week before he came into the hospital. Why then? He says that if he can't use the car, his wife and children certainly could. So he got a big car, just in case. In case of what? He doesn't answer, but says that he sold his business recently. What about the timing here, too? Just in case, again? He knew he'd be laid up for a while. Just in case, I persist. . . . The doctor doesn't hold out much hope, he thinks. Oh, I've had some x-ray treatments, but he dwindles off, shrugs slightly, as if he doesn't expect much. Now he seems to be talking in a whisper to himself. Maybe a month, probably much longer. I think that he'll be lucky to live through the next week. He puffs on a cigarette, puts it out, lights another. I watch, and think that his life is going up in smoke. A short smoke, then good night.

Returning to the car topic, I say that he evidently wanted to be sure that his family was well taken care of, by buying a big car and selling his business, regardless of the time ahead. He nods sadly. We both know. I feel sad. We sit silently, beyond words.

Debriefing spontaneously shifts back and forth, using both present and past tenses. It is ungrammatical, but emotionally very correct. Note that I used most of the information he gave in clarifying and providing collaborative relief. He did not need cooling off, but stirring up. Despite his reticence, customary coping came through, as well as the predominant concern: his family. He had taken steps to get ready cash for the family who would soon be on its own. The big, new car somehow symbolized the man, whom I kept thinking of as having much strength, now fading. It turned out that this was a correct surmise. But the significant feature of the debriefing is that even now I can reconstruct most of the session, though it occurred months ago. As I recall it well, I am also not far from feeling as I did when we sat silently together.

MORE ABOUT COUNTERCOPING

Interviewing and debriefing are only the outer edges of what goes on in countercoping. There is no step-by-step procedure, but the therapist can refer to Table 6 after debriefing and find the countercoping outcome or strategy that conforms most closely with what he or she did. Just as one cannot cope without a problem to contend with, countercoping needs another person. Each patient is unique. What he or she has to say is, therefore, worth heeding. This makes any intervention worthwhile, contributing bit by bit to forming a firm bulwark against storms of distress. The most important precept, however, is "Go with the flow, but don't drift." Not all things come to those who wait. Serendipity may be everywhere, but it is wise not to count on it, but to seek it out! Expectant behavior requires patience, and initiative. Spontaneity is a practiced art. Improvisation is to be cultivated. Wooden questions, dry routine, standard responses are dull and defeating.

As an example of more resourceful questioning with more productive results, let us first recall that patients with marital problems are at greater risk of alienation, over the course of illness. How can it be investigated?

Wrong

DR.: Have you had any trouble with your marriage?

PT.: No, my husband is a very good man. Why do you want to know? What has that to do with this lump?

The question calls for a yes or no answer, which would be hard to evaluate, regardless of how the patient responds. As it is, she is irritated. The question sounds as impertinent as if the doctor had asked, "Are you a good wife?" She is defensive, and asserts that her husband is a very good man, although that was not the question.

Few marriages are without troubles at times, and marital problems are irrelevant unless a connection with the illness can be shown.

Right

DR.: How helpful do you think your husband will be during this time, when you're likely to feel a little below par? I mean, judging by past experience, what do you expect?

PT.: He'll be all right, I guess. He's a very good man and a good father. Turns his paycheck over to me every week. I've really never been sick before, I mean like this. Always well. He doesn't like details. I don't think he's very sympathetic about illness, not that I need any sympathy. But maybe I'm afraid he'll think I should be exactly the same, up and doing, taking care of things. He wouldn't know how to wash a dish. How different will I be?

The questions are now acceptable and evocative. She does not accuse her husband of being excessively demanding, but expects that he will be somewhat inept and perhaps impatient with any limitation in her usual activity. Although she does not now claim that he is a good husband, she reveals a concern about coping, which is to be up and doing, taking care of things, not bothering her husband with details or decisions. Activity is more important than talk for them both. Marital problems, it seems, are not likely to be prominent. The clear, therapeutic implication, however, is that appropriate countercoping should seek a balance between convalescence and customary activity. The patient will, therefore, work out a schedule, consistent with being in charge of the household, minimizing the effect of treatment, but allowing for temporary limitations. Should a longer period of rest and rehabilitation be necessary, the husband might also be called in. Then one could tell how much change he tolerates.

This is a very simple example of how a good question discloses potential pressure points as well as customary coping strategies. The countercoping response is almost self-evident. But there are many other interchanges that are simply baffling.

> Doctor, I'm not sure what's happening, whether it's all real. Two weeks ago, I was working, feeling fine, not a care in the world. Now, here I am. I just can't believe that the x-ray showed a tumor in my chest. Could someone be wrong? Jesus! I lie awake at night, wondering. . . . I can't tell you about what. No! I'm not confused, that I'm sure about! I wake up, thinking about a TV show I saw, or just nothing at all. But I'm awake, not dreaming. I wish I could dream this up. Maybe I'll think about breakfast, or someone at work, or something someone said, or someone I knew years ago. I don't know. What difference does it make? I doze away for hours, without really sleeping. Yet I hate to wake up. I get angry at my doctor for no good reason, except that I'm here and he's there. My heart breaks. I feel for my poor wife. She brings me clean pajamas every day, and I couldn't care less. I pretend it's a bad dream, but I know that no one is sure of anything, even a bad dream. That's just words. Can anyone help me get over this cloud in my head? I doubt it. Sure, I'll take the treatment. What choice do I have? By the way, what did you say your name is?

No physician or consultant helps when he flings himself into despair along with the patient. He may, however, respond inappropriately, uttering a few inanities ("You'll feel better soon!"), and back out of the room. He will do better to make sense out of the patient's feelings of endangerment and annihilation. This patient is on the brink of confusion ("things have happened too fast, maybe they aren't real"), but at the moment he is simply very concerned and uncertain.

As so often happens, the reported interchange, fragmented and one-sided, makes more sense by reading it backwards, from the last question about my name to his initial uncertainty about reality. Asking for my name is not accidental. I regard it as an indirect request for help in clearing up the cloud in his head. He also needs strategic countercoping which establishes facts as presently understood, and restores a sense of time and options. Otherwise, he is a hapless victim, contending with unexpected, but threatening, external events. Asking who I am logically follows from his uncertainty about who he is and what he can expect.

In general, good countercoping mirrors the aims of good coping. The patient should be able to recast problems into solvable form, while preserving self-esteem. Because a patient ought to be an effective person in his or her own eyes, countercoping also respects reality testing. The original problem may be beyond options. But some choices are still available. These are consistent with how the patient coped before the illness descended. No patient should feel like a puppet manipulated by forces beyond comprehension.

Case 30   Frieda was a strong-willed, 69-year-old woman with an ovarian carcinoma who suddenly decided that she did not want to see her husband or five grown children. The family was dismayed, but Frieda was adamant. I was called in to consult because her attitude was so uncharacteristic that the physician thought she was becoming paranoid, or depressed, at the very least.

She had been told about the diagnosis and treatment very carefully and seemed to have understood and accepted the uncertainty. Nevertheless, she insisted that no one visit, because she would soon be home again. I wondered what one had to do with the other, since there was a gap in logic between the two statements, one of which justified the other in some way.

I learned that Frieda was an old-school matriarch who decided for the family what needed to be done, what was worth doing, and who should do it. The family acquiesced, and now felt that they had inadvertently made her angry. She was not, however, abrasively tyrannical or even very demanding. In fact, she knew they were all dependent on her, and took some of the blame. She was also aware of how distraught the family was about being kept from visiting.

The key problem came out when Frieda said that whenever her family visited, she began to cry, a most unusual display for her. She felt weak, miserable, and humiliated *because,* by crying, she let them down. Obviously, she also let herself down in some way. But she was very tired, and once felt very strong. She was tearful, when once everyone relied on her composure. Now she was uncertain, no longer knowing what to do or how to do what needed doing. So she sent the family away until she could regain her confidence. During a lengthy interview, Frieda never spoke about her illness except for its effect on the family and her own self-esteem.

Frieda did not want to see her family, and knew that it was not their fault, but a self-imposed withdrawal. She also reported ordering them, on more than one occasion, to be more independent! My countercoping target (or outcome) was to restore Frieda to the position she had held, namely, the supportive head of the family, while helping her toward emancipating the children, as surely they would want to be, and as surely as she professed wanting them to be.

Had she been in regular psychotherapy, a most unlikely supposition, she would have tried to run her own treatment. Now, however, she was almost flat on her back, facing prolonged treatment. More exactly, she had her back to the wall, finding it difficult to maintain her customary poise while depressed and tearful.

I advised that her most important decision was to acknowledge that she had needs too, and that she could allow her family to witness and share her sorrow. It was not a sign of weakness, but a chance to set another good example, as she always had. It would be good for them to know that even their strong mother could feel weak and worn out. Her tears meant sorrow, nothing more, and she was rightfully sad. I pointed out that true weakness would be to conceal her actual feelings. Permitting the family to visit and share would be a responsible act in that it showed confidence in them. It delegated authority by her choice, which she had, up until now, not done, except by telling others what to do. Letting them visit was a way of letting them go, which was an act of love. They could find independence by her consent, without giving her up. She could be more helpful than ever.

Several more days elapsed. I saw her once more. Frieda listened, but added very little. When my ideas finally seemed to be hers or had sufficient impact, she allowed the family to visit, and was no longer tearful. Her weakness improved. Whether my countercoping had an effect, or Frieda simply waited until she regained composure, neither of us shall ever know.

THE LEAST POSSIBLE CONTRIBUTION

Countercoping is really a form of "palliation" which is not confined to patients beyond cure. In Frieda's case, the problem that caused her to withdraw was confronted (Cope 6) and interpreted in an acceptable form (Cope 7). Then she could act according to her own best self-concept and reality testing, without construing weakness as deplorable.

Palliation means covering up, but I define palliation as a guise in which unacceptable facts become *copeful.* Frieda would have balked, but I simply told her what to do. However, she accepted the opportunity to assert herself as a good mother on whom the children, and her husband, could rely.

Other cancer patients need much less. Just knowing that they have acceptable options is often enough. What was the patient like before the illness took over? This will offer us a clue about what to do and how coping should work out. Only a very few patients seek miracles in untested remedies, which, of course, is still another option.

It is only important to protect patients from imprudent behavior and unscrupulous exploitation. Is the proposal consistent with safe conduct? Is the price more than its value? The philosophy that there is nothing to lose, so why not try anything, is misleading, at best. Preterminal patients, for example, may lose a chance for a comparatively serene accommodation, sharing penultimate events with those who mean most, or at least having an option to do whatever they wish. No one need be demoralized by a chronic illness, or be asked to endure a meaningless tragedy, feeling that he or she is less than a full person. This would only compound the tragedy.

Countercoping can be vexing, frustrating, imprecise, and even, at times, very rewarding. It is never contentious, although resentful, endangered patients take out feelings on whoever is at hand. The effect of countercoping is seldom demonstrated forcefully. Clarification and control, collaboration, directed relief, and reduction of emotional extremes gently tend to flow together, just as perception, will, emotion, and behavior belong to a functional unit designed to bring about wished-for change. Countercoping is not very drastic or dramatic. However, its effectiveness is probably proportional to its spontaneity, provided that the therapist is emphatic and empathic enough to modulate his or her own expectations and feelings.[10] A simple clarification, a mild confrontation, or even more vigorous insistence upon postponing a critical, but imprudent decision may be more helpful than trying to initiate far-reaching, overweening programs that the very nature of the medical plight will not permit. Too much ambition, like too much pessimism, carries its own defeat and destruction.

I have repeatedly emphasized that a little goes a long way, especially when countercoping enters into the flow of the predicament. Hence, I advocate a principle called the *least possible contribution.* It does not mean doing as little as possible. People seem to learn that without being taught. The least possible contribution is one with the least strain, but has the best chance of making a difference, however small. Then, having made such a contribution, another and still another can be added until something quite substantial and unanticipated results. Morale seems to be better, distress is less, and coping is more explicit and effective. After all, the primary purpose of countercoping, with its several outcomes, is to do for cancer patients with emotional distress what patients who cope well seem to do by themselves.

REFERENCES

1 Hackett, T. , and N. Cassem, (eds.), *MGH Handbook of Liaison Psychiatry,* C. V. Mosby Company, St. Louis, 1979.
2 Hackett, T., "The Psychiatrist: In the Mainstream or on the Banks of Medicine," *American Journal of Psychiatry,* **134**(4): 432–434, April 1977.
3 Dunbar, F., *Psychosomatic Diagnosis,* Paul B. Hoeber, Inc., New York and London, 1943.
4 LeShan, L., *You Can Fight for Your Life: Emotional Factors in the Causation of Cancer,* M. Evans and Company, Inc., New York, 1977.
5 Fox, B., *Premorbid Psychological Factors as Related to Incidence of Cancer,* National Cancer Institute Publication, Bethesda, Md., 1976.
6 Maccoby, E., and N. Maccoby, "The Interview: A Tool of Social Science," in Lindzey, G. (ed.), *Handbook of Social Psychology,* vol. I, Addison-Wesley Publishing Company, Inc., Cambridge, Mass., 1954, pp. 449–487.
7 Deutsch, F., and W. Murphy, *The Clinical Interview: A Method of Teaching Associative Exploration,* International Universities Press, Inc., New York, 1955.
8 Rogers, C., "Client-centered Psychotherapy," in A. Freedman, H. Kaplan, and B. Sadock (eds.), *Comprehensive Textbook of Psychiatry II,* The Williams & Wilkins Company, Baltimore, 2d ed., 1975, vol. II, chap. 30, 3, pp. 1831–1842.
9 Bird, B., *Talking with Patients,* 2d ed., J. B. Lippincott Company, Philadelphia and Toronto, 1973.
10 Lewis, J., "Practicum in Attention to Affect: A Course for Beginning Psychotherapists," *Psychiatry,* **37**: 109–113, 1974.

Cancer, Morale, and the Human Predicament

VOCATIONAL MORALE

One of the hazards of working in health care, education, social services, and similar occupations is losing vocational morale. The drain and strain may be too much. Some talented people drop into the role of a functionary; filling forms, handing out medications, snipping lesions become all the same. Cancer care, in particular, requires a high order of competence, devotion, and morale just to cope with seemingly endless problems. True professionals must get along on very thin rations at times—occasional cures, partial remissions, symptom-free intervals, and appreciative patients. Sometimes, what is needed is to transcend tragedy and keep working. The rigors of coping with problems that cannot wholly be dispelled invite a sense of failure, which should be resisted. Limitations in recovery potential, as well as in what we can do, require limitless morale. But cope we must. There is no alternative, other than capitulation. Regardless of accomplishments, our vocation has an infinitely receding horizon. The number of problems remaining unsolved always demands performance beyond present capabilities.

119

Coping with cancer, whether as patient, professional, or both, means more than coping with a chronic disease. It is coping with the human predicament, which is misery surrounded by misfortune. Cancer can be an inexhaustible, relentless, and resourceful foe. Without strong vocational morale, we are tempted to play it safe, without offering safe conduct (Chapter 2). Whatever strengthens our morale, however, fortifies the morale of people we deal with. Reciprocally, a cancer patient who copes exceedingly well replenishes our efforts with a sense of purpose.

DEMORALIZATION AND DESPAIR

It is a revealing commentary on our predicament to realize that there are dozens of words which refer to shades and qualities of sadness, dejection, depression, and hopelessness, and very few words in our language for well-being. Eskimos, I am told, have many words to describe snow. I assume that they have little need to describe green grass. Evidently, we need to recognize many varieties of demoralization and despair because such feelings are so prevalent in daily life. Ordinary, tolerable, comfortable well-being is certainly not conveyed by "happiness," as I mentioned earlier. Good copers might even feel rebuked, if someone called them "happy." "Normothymia" is as silly a neologism as "eupepsia." Both terms sound like diseases looking for symptoms. But the implication is that our prevailing predicament finds us immersed in abundant ill-feelings, not well-being. It is therefore fair to assume that normal morale is generally rather feeble and transitory, and that demoralization and despair are more common than their opposites.

Despair, as I pointed out in Chapter 5, is at the core of vulnerability. It is found amid apathy, strong denial, alienation, annihilation, and endangerment. It can also appear in much milder forms, such as when someone feels embittered, imposed upon, victimized, relentlessly rushed, excessively fatigued, anxious, and realizes that we are all too mortal, too soon. Despair is no stranger in cancer care, especially when shortcomings are considered to be sins, limitations are failures, and error is evil. If this occurs, the professional is suffering from vocational demoralization and despair.

CANCER AND SOCIETY

In a way, malignancy is a form of malevolence. Cancer is not so unique among diseases, if it is only considered a biological problem. But, publicity notwithstanding, cancer is more than a group of diseases which have largely baffled investigators. Cancer is still, in many circles, a taboo topic, surrounded by superstitions and death imagery.

Are there other diseases in which the question of withholding information is ever discussed? For what other disease do we incessantly search for synonyms, instead of calling it by the right name? The often cold, penetrating anguish of a cancer patient has a special significance. It threatens morale more than other maladies. Conversely, the cured cancer patient is treated almost reverently, like a hero who has triumphantly come through something dreadful. The cured cancer patient not only becomes an automatic authority on how to cope, but feels entitled to evangelize.

Cancer is also symbolic of contemporary social ills. In biblical times, the symbolic disease was leprosy. Later, it was plague, then tuberculosis and syphilis. All of these diseases, long before the discovery of bacteria and protozoa, carried a fatal taint, an aura of accursedness that required some holy intervention to cure. Meanwhile, victims were shunned, segregated, often exiled. We may be somewhat more temperate today, but cancer is still thought of, by some, as a dirty, deadly disease, and its victims may be set apart. There is a bigotry about cancer that well-intentioned, medical abolitionists have not eradicated. Cancer patients have been refused jobs, insurance, housing, and so forth, regardless of their medical status. While cancer patients may claim that they once had cancer, when asked months later, others are more cautious. It might come back. Cure is a word to be used with care. Only in the recent past has medicine become somewhat demythologized. But cancer carries its own mythology.

Solzhenitsyn's *Cancer Ward* and Mann's *Magic Mountain* use cancer and tuberculosis, respectively, as metaphors for the human predicament. Patients are players who perform their private roles against a backdrop of incorrigible disease or fateful tragedy. I have known cancer specialists who were advised by mentors to avoid the field, lest their careers be ruined by what seems to be inherent frustration and defeat. Of course, psychiatrists are accustomed to this attitude. The attitude of outsiders toward psychiatry and cancerology is somewhat similar. Both represent risky specialties which are both praiseworthy and perhaps nonproductive, almost aboriginal specialties. Practitioners are, therefore, stigmatized, whether positively, with admiration and respect, or negatively, as hard-working but somewhat ineffectual. Medicine may not be a magical profession any longer, but there is hardly any question but that morale in cancer work is an everpresent issue, perhaps because we secretly yearn for magical solutions, and, of course, are destined to disappointment.

PROTAGORAS AND THE PROBLEM OF MORALE

Protagoras, a fifth-century B.C. philosopher, is chiefly remembered for two comments, both quoted out of context.[1] Nevertheless, his thoughts are pertinent for our central question of how to cope with cancer.

> With regard to the gods, I cannot feel sure that they are or are not, nor what they are like. There are many things that hinder sure knowledge, such as the obscurity of the subject, and the brevity of human life.

Man is the measure of all things, of things that are as they are, and of things that are not because they are not.

From this distance in time, I feel sure that Protagoras would allow me to paraphrase him according to our own culture and problems. After all, it is impossible to speak for all ages and eras, to stand outside of where we are now, or to examine the human predicament with total objectivity. We are not only products of our times, but its prisoners as well. Many things hinder sure knowledge. Mysteries in this world are not necessarily common knowledge for the next. We can only live in one world; the rest is speculation. About the gods, he knew as little as I. He relied on human understanding, despite fallibility and obstacles. We have nothing more.

Man is the measure of all things. I understand this in two ways: (1) Man is the measure by which all things are judged, that is, according to their human consequences; (2) man is the measurer of all things that are, as well as those that are wholly conjectural.

Measurement is what science is all about. Meaning is what philosophy is all about. Man's plight in trying to measure the meaning of man is filled with paradoxes and ambiguities. Too much information; too little wisdom. Too many instruments; too little creativity. Too much conformity; too little compassion. We are numbed by numbers, and do not know what those numbers mean in terms of human existence. We are dazzled by sheer speed, without knowing where we are heading. Violence, poverty, pollution, war, famine, disease, pestilence are not merely horsemen of the Apocalypse. They are an entire cavalry, pitted against humanity. *Cancer symbolizes them all.* As physician and psychiatrist, I often ponder whether survival is worth the effort, especially for certain cancer patients or those psychiatric patients who may suffer even more. This question is epitomized in the incessant struggle between cancer and morale.

MORALE AND QUALITY OF LIFE

Physical health is an opportunity, not a given right or privilege. It should be protected and even treasured. No one knows this better than a chronic cancer patient who is often asked to forfeit quality of life for uncertain survival. Chemotherapy or radiation may add extra time, perhaps even unlimited survival, but often at an enormous price. Chemotherapy can cause vomiting, gastrointestinal ulceration, neuritis, hair loss, and many other toxic aberrations that further compromise and impoverish existence. Radiation often drains the cancer patient until it reaches a bone-deep fatigue that seldom relents, and burns away not just tissues, but the will to live.

Of course, I am not referring to cancer patients with an excellent chance of cure or remission. The trade-in value for its price in troublesome side effects is a bargain. Rather, I mean patients beyond substantial help, for whom chemotherapy, radiation, and surgery inflict other diseases, sometimes more dreadful, debasing, and deadlier than the original cancer.

Conscientious physicians recognize the moral dilemma, including long-term consequences of treatment that so often is cavalierly recommended. These doctors encourage patients to make an enlightened choice, knowing that they must also offer safe conduct, standing by with full support, instead of vanishing into thickets of statistics when problems pile up.

Not every physician is so conscientious, nor is every patient able to make an intelligent decision. Uncertainty and ambiguity move at an equal pace. Indeed, some patients prefer to have the decision taken away (Cope 14) in order to suppress anxiety (Cope 4). Other patients agree to desperation medicine, because it is a kind of Hobson's choice. Nevertheless, to have an option or a range of choices, whether exercised or not, is at least symbolic recognition of the importance of morale in affording significance to survival, which also means good quality of life.

The facile, contemporary phrase "quality of life" is still a puzzle. Practically everyone seems to know what it means, but no one can adequately define, classify, or measure it. Certainly it is better to be healthy than sick, better to walk than be confined to a wheelchair, better to be solvent than on welfare, better to breathe clean air than carcinogens. But as we go on, comparing the better with the worse, choices become more uncertain and dependent on values we hold. What "quality of life" means and is measured against as a general proposition remains elusive.

Quality of life can be divided into two main considerations:

1 General factors pertaining to society and the environment
2 Subjective factors relating to the significance of the individual

General factors include problems of population, poverty, health, energy, war, ignorance, bigotry, crime, ecology, and so forth, all social ills. Subjective factors are those that largely contribute to individual well-being and morale. Obviously, the two overlap, but quality of life is not completely determined by external calamities or noxious circumstances.

Subjective factors which contribute to well-being and morale are not the same as those that decide how long one lives. This is quantity of life, not quality. Significant survival, or an acceptable quality of life, requires options, respect, reasonable security, and a sense of living up to potential or within the scope of what is esteemed. According to some, medicine aims to keep people alive as long as possible, and as young as possible. This is because contemporary values decree that old age is a social ill and an inexorable disease that overtakes even the healthiest, and impoverishes quality of life.[2] If so, then growing older would be a menace. It may well be for some, damaging the individual's special significance and contributing the stigma of advancing years to the other general hazards of being alive.

In its subjective sense, not even the most ardent, eugenically minded practitioner would argue that good quality of life should be limited to the young in body or to the physically healthy, who need it least. Quality of life ought to come in all sizes for all people, including those who are growing older or have a chronic illness, such as cancer. Consternation about cancer and its consequences urges a somewhat antievolutionary slogan: not just survival of the fittest, but survival of the sickest, too, as long and as significantly as possible.[3] The hinge that separates general and special factors in quality of life is fastened to sturdy morale. Regardless of how well-off one is with respect to the environment and society, without morale and inner resources there is only anonymity, apathy, anger, and agony.

MORALE AND CANCER

In cancer, as with everything else, significant survival depends on how we would like to be and be seen when at our best. Belief that our life is worth living comes from realizing that our "best" conforms, more often than not, to our standards, otherwise known as an "ego ideal."[4] It is not, by any means, an ideal ego, conceived by mixing morals with a special brand of perfection. The ego ideal ensures survival on a reasonably high level of competence, with tolerable complaints, and a substantial residue of coping capacity. For the very sick or disabled, the ego ideal is necessarily a compromise between what is desirable and deplorable. But it still seeks to fit the person and plight together, with a certain harmonious acceptance. Regardless of the predicament, therefore, morale is self-esteem in action.

If there were a sure cure for cancer in all its forms, this discussion about morale would be superfluous. But since coping and vulnerability take place along a continuum of disability from none to almost total, morale assessment is a necessary aspect of comprehensive cancer care. Disability itself, however, is not a reliable measure of morale, any more than the size of the tumor measures the capacity to cope.

Freedom to exercise options coherently according to a personal standard of excellence is a hallmark of "man the measurer." In some situations, what one chooses is a moral act because its consequences are visualized as good or bad. William James proposed that we use group standards of excellence to divert socially destructive behavior into channels for productive, praiseworthy purposes.[5] These he called "moral equivalents." For the individual, moral equivalents would entitle a person to say, "This is me at my best."

Just as a piece of granite represents a potential work of art, a moral equivalent symbolizes human possibility. To be able to authenticate oneself in action requires a standard of excellence. Thus, a cancer patient who preserves personal responsibility, regardless of disease and ramifications, acquires a state of excellence which we admire and would emulate. But it is less a moral act or equivalent than one in which morale shines forth, illuminating and invigorating, in turn, our vocational morale.

Morale, a global sense of well-being and self-esteem, means more than high motivation, elevated mood, or moral behavior. As Allport demonstrated, self-authentication does not come easily.[6] Self-esteem is not only very fragile, but needs renewal. Morale, which is the private, subjective side of quality of life, is a much broader concept than morality, and one should not be confused with the other.

For the purpose of contending with cancer, I find that three components of morale are most important. These are (1) morale equivalents, (2) effective coping, and (3) self-awareness, a special kind of consciousness.

Morale Equivalents   No one ever became "ethical" just by being told to behave, reading uplifting books, or knowing that it is better to lead another kind of life. No one ever developed morale in this way, either. Admonitions, precepts, advice, and inspiring examples of morality or morale are quickly forgotten. For every moral directive about how to think or behave, there is an equal and opposite imperative or prohibition. Therefore, I deem it wise to leave categorical rules for others, provided that I am not required to practice what they preach. Meanwhile, personal morale helps any one of us practice what we believe is best for us.

The concept of equivalents is not new in medicine. Common illnesses are replaced by less common, but equally diagnostic indicators. The equivalent is a guise which reveals more than it conceals. Nevertheless, it requires a certain acumen to recognize an equivalent, and to know what it means. Morale equivalents are *token acts* representing the ego ideal in action, such that the part stands for the whole. Acts of self-esteem in purposeful survival are emblematic of someone at his or her best.

A significant act which typifies morale presents itself not by design, but spontaneously, just-so, as if there were no other choice, because this is what one is and wants to be. It is, of course, impossible always to be at one's best, or to behave consistently according to ideal standards. Nevertheless, scattered morale equivalents help to generate further acts of the same high quality. When, for example, a husband asks how he should treat his ailing wife, the proper answer is, "Just as you would when *you* are at your best." Unwittingly, the husband has raised a very real question about his morale. It is not a moral or ethical question. Understanding this, we respond with a directive designed to fortify his morale, despite trying circumstances.

Morale equivalents are exemplified in daily life by physicians, clergy, nurses, social workers, teachers, and by conscientious workers of all kinds. Morale may be spontaneous, but it also needs practice, not preachment. By the same tokens, these people often lapse or are delinquent in practicing morale. Adherence to high standards of competence and compassion is not a matter of resolve, external codes, contracts, or impersonal arrangements. Again, it is something that happens, possibly because there is no real alternative. For example, in 1972, the American Hospital Association adopted a statement of principles, or "Bill of Rights," for patient care.[7] However, it listed only what good professionals try to do, anyway, just-so, because another course would be unthinkable, or at least abrasively inconsistent with morale standards. Any Bill of Rights is the outcome of good practice, not a set of directives, laws, or incentives. It is a proclamation of coping and countercoping excellence.

One morale equivalent encourages another. The "befitting" act helps the fit between a patient and the plight. For instance, a mother of small children will spontaneously consider the impact of illness on her family, such that coping with anticipated problems represents a morale equivalent, namely, as she would be or become at her best. Frieda (Case 30) is a good example of restorative morale, that is, coping assisted by appropriate countercoping.

Effective Coping   Vulnerability exposes a fault in morale; effective coping strengthens morale. It is, of course, unreasonable and foolhardy to expect permanent, once-and-for-all coping effectiveness for the healthy, let alone the ill or infirm. Patients who say, "I can manage," may well do so, but a substantial part of managing is to know when and whom to ask for help. Effective coping is part of morale because we need a self-confirmatory test of competence and purpose to carry us from one problem to the next. That is but one reason why, throughout this book, I have emphasized the *enduring and incessant* process of coping, which is, at best, only exemplified by general coping strategies. If there is any purpose in being alive or surviving well, it is to cope effectively with problems that present themselves, in order to deal with the next problem, and sustain our morale.

Self-awareness   The never-ending task of coping, correcting, coping, and correcting again and again, until this or that problem recedes, requires a lasting sense of personal awareness or identity. This is the tenacious "I" amid the sights, sounds, smells, touches, and coming-and-goings of others. Self-awareness is to be conscious of what is real or uppermost—"things that are as they are and things that are not because they are not." What is real is real for me, and what is real for me is real.[4] This injunction has a stark validity for the cancer patient or someone for whom that patient is very precious. To be sick and sick at heart have much in common, and both can equally erode morale. Cancer changes reality, poignantly confirming that we are all enclosed in a little compartment that makes communication all but impossible. At moments of vulnerability, cancer patients sometimes become "self-aware" for the very first time. They have lived long without understanding the underlying denominator of much that happens. Whether self-esteem, the world, or the body and organs therein deteriorates, man is the measure of all things. Whatever takes place happens also to thee.

Self-awareness is to be conscious of consciousness for a purpose, even while thinking about other things. Conversely, that most misused and misunderstood concept called consciousness means to be aware *of* something *for* some action, *as* someone special. For the cancer patient awareness of meaningless islands of ill-formed yet voracious cells within can damage morale, because it separates what one is from what one could be in the here-and-now. Nevertheless, by heeding such self-awareness, it may be possible to fuse consciousness of sickness with the just-so of morale. These islands are not, after all, the mainland of morale, where we really live. Morale is tested by how well ambiguity, threat, paradox and plurality are tolerated. However, when we realize that what we do makes sense only by anticipating consequences, without undue alarm, then self-awareness can become a strength. Morale then is a vision guiding how we cope, and generating hope.

IS COPING ENOUGH?

I do not expect that these philosophical ruminations about morale and the human predicament will, in themselves, prove much immediate consolation for cancer patients, friends, families, or medical professionals. Few others care. Nevertheless, all of us search for remedies that will provide a structure and reason for coping, instead of capitulation. Regular medical treatment, rehabilitation, and a host of other factors pertaining to quality of life should reinforce, not undermine morale. Good quality of life, essential to the cancer patient, as well as others, depends on knowing what works and what does not work under various circumstances. That sense of hope and direction constitutes morale.

Is coping enough? Not until the enigma of cancer is solved can we dispense with coping. But is science enough, without considering the problems and personality of afflicted people who seek a life they can live with? I truly support the popular refrain "Cancer can be cured." But I also know that it applies only to some types of cancer under special circumstances. "Cancer can be cured" is still a program and a promise. Not everyone now qualifies for cured cancer clubs. Coping well requires that we recognize the disparity between what one wants, and what can be expected in the here-and-now. Coping effectively is not always the same as coping successfully.

Myths are frequently our masters. One need not be mortified by failures, shortcomings, errors, or supercede them with demoralization and despair. Despite its limitations, morale always offers a chance at self-renewal.

In the light of history and futurity, I obviously feel an affinity with the perplexed Protagoras. Man is the measure, but how shall man be measured? My visceral answer is that man measures himself by and through his morale under trying conditions, such as in the existential plight of cancer. Morale, therefore, can be its own justification.

We rue the brevity of life, the obscurity of the subject, being born too soon, and having no gods to represent our case. But morale equivalents, good coping, and self-awareness about excellence in dealing with human problems have a way of persisting, regardless of the progress of science or the deception encouraged by fads and fashions of our times. These human issues will probably be just as relevant 2500 years from now. And perhaps by that time, cancer will only be a topic for antiquarians to ponder.

REFERENCES

1 De Santillana, G., *The Origins of Scientific Thought,* "Man, the Difficult Measure," Mentor Books, New York, 1961, chap. 10, pp. 168–184.
2 Butler, R., and M. Lewis, *Aging and Mental Health,* C. V. Mosby, New York, 1973.
3 Weisman, A., "The Psychiatrist and the Inexorable," in H. Feifel (ed.), *New Meanings of Death,* McGraw-Hill Book Company, New York, 1977, pp. 107–122.
4 Weisman, A., *The Existential Core of Psychoanalysis: Reality Sense and Responsibility,* Little, Brown and Company, Boston, 1965.
5 James, W., "The Moral Equivalent of War," in R. Perry (ed.), *Essays on Faith and Morals,* Meridian Books, New American Library, New York, 1962, pp. 311–328.
6 Allport, G., *Becoming: Basic Considerations for a Psychology of Personality,* Terry Lectures, Yale University Press, New Haven and London, 1955.
7 Curran, W. J., "The Patient's Bill of Rights Becomes Law," *New England Journal of Medicine,* **290:** 32–33, Jan. 3, 1974.

BIBLIOGRAPHY

Annals of New York Academy of Sciences: "Psychophysiological Aspects of Cancer," vol. 125, pp. 773–1055, 1966, E. Weyer (ed.).

———: "Second Conference on Psychophysiological Aspects of Cancer," vol. 164, pp. 307–634, 1969, M. Krauss, P. Albertson, and C. Bahnson (eds.).

———: "Care of Patients with Fatal Illness," vol. 164, pp. 635–896, 1969, M. Krauss and L. White (eds.).

Coelho, G., D. Hamburg, and J. Adams (eds.), *Coping and Adaptation*, Basic Books, Inc., New York, 1974.

Cullen, Jr., B. Fox, and R. Isom (eds.), *Cancer: The Behavioral Dimensions*, Raven Press, New York, 1976.

Feifel, H. (ed.), *New Meanings of Death*, McGraw-Hill Book Company (Blakiston Publication), New York, 1977.

Holland, J., "Psychologic Aspects of Cancer," in J. Holland and E. Frei (eds.), *Cancer Medicine*, Lea & Febiger, Philadelphia, 1973, pp. 991–1021.

Murphy, L., and A. Moriarty, *Vulnerability, Coping, & Growth from Infancy to Adolescence*, Yale University Press, New Haven and London, 1976.

Weisman, A., and J. Worden, *Coping and Vulnerability in Cancer Patients: A Research Report*, Shea Bros., Cambridge, Mass., 1977.

Index

Index